AROMA FREEDOM

Break Through to Your New Life with Aroma and Neuroscience

Dr. Benjamin Perkus

Aroma Freedom

Break Through to Your New Life with Aroma and Neuroscience

DEDICATION

To my wife Elaine, my spiritual and personal companion throughout all of our many journeys in the realms of teaching, healing, and living. Thank you for continuing to expect the best from me and supporting my quest for better ways of helping others.

To my daughter Eyana, your belief in my abilities to detect and fix problems has inspired me to believe in myself even more, and to create something to help the generations to come.

To Gary Young and all of the members of Young Living Essential Oils, the community of innovative, caring, and open souls who seek a better life has been a source of learning and growth for over 20 years.

Finally, to my past and future students of Aroma Freedom. It is through conversations with you that these techniques have been created, refined, tested, and finally brought into the world at large. This book is dedicated to everyone who has been placed on the path of personal and professional development and who finds in these pages some inspiration to dive more deeply into the human adventure!

"Determine that the thing can and shall be done and then...
find the way."

- *Abraham Lincoln*

CONTENTS

Endorsement from Jack Canfield

Coauthor of the #1 *New York Times bestselling Chicken Soup for the Soul® series* and *The Success Principles™: How to Get from Where You Are to Where You Want to Be*

"If you are looking to release limiting beliefs that are holding you back (many of which you are not even aware you have), I highly recommend Dr. Benjamin Perkus and the Aroma Freedom Technique.

I have done several sessions with Dr. Perkus that turned out to be major breakthroughs for me in terms of identifying, releasing and replacing several limiting beliefs that I wasn't even aware I had and that were stopping me from moving forward on things that were important to me and my business.

And because I recommended that some of my Canfield trainers study with him and become certified AFT practitioners, I have also experienced several sessions with some of my trainers who became certified. Every time I have had a significant breakthrough.

While the work is very deep and powerful, the process itself has always been surprisingly easy. The brilliant use of essential oils along with the 12-step process that Dr. Perkus created makes the process amazingly easy to do. I am still amazed at how quickly and easily the transformation occurred. And the best part is the results have been permanent."

INTRODUCTION

How to Read This Book

—⸙⸎⸙⸎⸙—

This book describes a new technique that represents an integration of psychology and aromatherapy. By using the sense of smell as part of the emotional clearing process, you can bypass your conscious mind and achieve fast and permanent results in how you view yourself and the world.

The technique is based on years of clinical experience, academic research, and observation of what works to set people free emotionally so that they can pursue their goals and dreams. I have taught this technique to thousands of people in the last 8 years and am now making it available to a wider audience.

I wrote this book for two reasons:

1. People are suffering because they are held back by inner obstacles (anxiety, depression, guilt, regret, worry, loneliness, procrastination) and because they don't know how to tackle the outer obstacles (taking inspired action, building success in work and relationships). In this book, you will find some powerful and simple tools you can use on yourselves and your loved ones to get you on track towards reaching your goals and dreams. You will find that you will feel more hopeful about your future, and you will become free of distressing memories that have haunted you from the past.

2. People who are therapists, counselors, coaches, and healing arts professionals know that helping others can be challenging and are always looking for more effective ways to get their clients un-stuck and moving in the right direction. If you are a helping professional, you will find here a refreshingly simple, yet scientifically grounded, set of techniques that can be used to enhance your effectiveness and potentially transform your practice. By combining the ancient art of aromatherapy with the latest advances in psychology and neuroscience, you will be able to offer your clients a cutting-edge approach that is gentle yet profound. Most importantly, it can be integrated with the style of therapy or coaching that you currently utilize in a way that both you and your clients will find enjoyable and rewarding.

I am going to be transparent with you throughout this book as to what you can and cannot accomplish with this method. As a self-care tool, it can help you to shift your emotional state and boost your motivation in many surprising ways - yet it is not a replacement for seeking a qualified professional if you are having trouble functioning on your own. As an addition to a professional practice, it may greatly accelerate your results - yet it will not be the right tool for every client, or for every problem. By the end of this book, you will have a much better idea of the range of problems that Aroma Freedom can address.

If you want to use the processes described in this book on yourself, family, or friends, you will learn enough in this book to begin transforming how you react to everyday stressors and to change how you approach the situations in your life. You may begin to feel more empowered and hopeful about reaching your goals. If you are a healing professional, I also suggest starting with yourself until you become comfortable with the processes. If you like the results you are getting, contact us to learn about our professional trainings.

I have structured this book as follows:

First, you will learn the story behind Aroma Freedom – how I discovered it in 2016 as a novel way to dissolve negative thoughts, feelings, and memories using essential oils. The results were so astonishingly gentle and powerful, that people immediately began to ask to become certified in the method. I learned right away to use the process on myself to help me "grow into" the rapidly growing online academy that I was creating. I discovered that, by using the technique daily, I could stay ahead of the learning curve that I suddenly needed to climb, and how I could help others do this as well.

Next, you will see the stories of some of the people who have been helped through Aroma Freedom in many areas of life, including:

- Freedom of Expression
- Freedom from Negative Moods, Behaviors, or Habits
- Freedom from Painful Memories
- Freedom from Powerlessness and Victimization
- Freedom from Paralysis and Self-Doubt
- Freedom of Self-Forgiveness + Inner Guidance
- Freedom to Help Others

You will also see some of the data we collected on how effective Aroma Freedom is to help people feel more confident and hopeful in reaching their goals.

We will explore the concept of personal and professional freedom and will do some self-assessments to see how well you are faring in both your emotional freedom and, if you are a professional, in your therapy, coaching, or healing practice. This will include things like satisfying employment and relationships, ability to feel the full range of human emotions without judgment, and the ability to help yourself or others to overcome traumatic memories.

Before going into the technique itself, we will also discuss why freedom and fulfillment are so difficult to attain. As highly evolved/divinely created human beings, we have the tendency to try to solve our problems using only our logic and our conscious minds...but often, that is not where the source of the problem comes from. We also can spend time endlessly theorizing about what to do to feel better, when in reality, the solution will come by cutting through all of the complexity and getting to the root of the matter. Finally, we discuss how important it is to develop a solid foundation for change before just trying to start a new habit or belief system without clearing away the old. All these problems are addressed by Aroma Freedom – because the sense of smell bypasses the conscious mind and stimulates the brain areas that will lead to intuitive problem solving, emotional peace, and unstoppable motivation.

The connection between the sense of smell and stimulation of memory is well documented – just think of how smelling fresh baked bread takes you back to your grandmother's kitchen. In my first book, "The Aroma Freedom Technique," I touched on this phenomenon and why it occurs. In the current book, I will take you much deeper into the science of memory as it relates to smell.

You will learn about the power of the sense of smell to quickly shift your mental and emotional state. Animals use their sense of smell to find food, attract mates, and avoid predators. People use their noses for all these things and more, as we shall see.

Since ancient times, people have enhanced their living environments with the beautiful scents of flowers, incense, spices, and perfumes. Additionally, scent has been used in places of worship to evoke a feeling of reverence and peace. This is because the sense of smell is anatomically designed to immediately stimulate the limbic system of the brain, which is responsible for processing emotions and memories.

I will show you which scents I have discovered to be the most effective at shifting the mental stress connected to upsetting memories, and how alternating through a few basic but powerful types of scent can create optimal results during the sessions.

We will look at the neuroscience of Memory Reconsolidation as the well-researched basis through which Aroma Freedom works. By understanding this natural brain process, we can learn to dissolve not just long-standing painful memories, but also to stop current stressors and even future worries from becoming fixated in our minds and emotions.

Memory Reconsolidation is an important advance in the understanding of how to resolve emotional problems, because it shows us how to become free of these problems in a way that we do not have to continually fight against our tendencies. When a memory is reconsolidated, it actually changes our brain structure in such a way that the old information is rewritten and the newer, more functional thoughts, feelings, and tendencies can be easily implemented.

I will give tips for self-management of moods, motivation, focus, communication, and personal as well as professional achievement. Learning how to quickly shift your mood and emotional reactions with Aroma Freedom will empower you to transform how you approach the stressors and problems in your life.

We will discuss some of the biggest problems that therapists and coaches run into when working with their clients, and how Aroma Freedom can help. In fact, one of the biggest problems for people working in those fields is burnout - not having anything left to give, especially when clients are struggling with difficult problems such as current or past trauma, hopelessness, or crippling anxiety and paralysis. Aroma Freedom offers therapists and coaches new tools that are easy to use, powerful, and very gentle. Clients love it as well because it does not require them to keep telling their stories over and over, and because it helps them feel better fast.

At the heart of the Aroma Freedom approach is the unique way in which we integrate the realms of Psychology and Aromatherapy. We use specific questions to identify the core "stuck points" in the mind that are related to the problem at hand. Then, when our client is in that awareness, we bring in the power of aroma. **This has a uniquely disruptive effect on consciousness, such that it enables the mind to completely restructure how a memory, situation, or future concern is perceived.** When we change perception in this way, we alter our very approach to reality itself. What had seemed hopeless is suddenly hopeful, what was once experienced as painful and heavy is now light and filled with possibility and meaning.

We will then discuss the 6 techniques of Aroma Freedom in detail. I will show you exactly how to do each of the 6 techniques both on yourself and on others. I will give tips for success so that you can avoid some of the common pitfalls that happen when first learning and mastering the processes. We will also review when the best time is to use each technique, as well as when you need to refer someone (or yourself!) to a qualified Mental Health Practitioner.

Finally, I will introduce you to a way to jump-start your results with Aroma Freedom so that you can quickly experience some of its many benefits. I will also connect you with bonus material and videos so that you can take your experience deeper, even as you are still learning.

This all may seem like a lot, but really, the entirety of this book may be summed up in these three points:

Point #1: The recent discovery of Aroma Freedom allows for a much faster, gentler, and more precise clearing of the emotional problems that beset almost everyone.

Point #2: Aroma Freedom can be used as a self-care modality to experience greater freedom and results in life, or it can be integrated into current models of therapy and coaching in a way that enhances their effectiveness.

Point #3: Aroma Freedom is founded based on the integration of the two disciplines of Psychology and Aromatherapy. The process works through the neuro-scientifically validated process of Memory Reconsolidation.

Aroma Freedom represents the culmination of over 20 years of research and practice using the latest breakthroughs in traditional as well as energy psychology, and aromatherapy. It has changed my life, and the lives of thousands of people since it was created in 2016, and it is my hope that it will change yours as well.

Then, if you are inspired to want to help others, you can reach out to my team to learn more about becoming a Certified Aroma Freedom Practitioner. This training is available to lay people and professionals alike. To learn more about the training and how to get started, just book a call with us at: www.aromafreedom.com/call

Remember, to use these techniques effectively, you will need specific essential oils - see the Appendix to learn what these are, why we use them, and how to get them so you can have your own breakthroughs right away!

NOTE: Part 1 of this book contains many stories, case studies, explanations, and questions designed to inspire you to see how Aroma Freedom can help you. I encourage you to read these stories and engage with these questions.. However, if you are eager to jump right in and try the techniques, you are welcome to jump ahead to part 2, especially Chapter 8 and beyond. You can always go back and read part 1 later. Enjoy!

To your success and freedom,
Dr. Benjamin Perkus.

Part 1:
FOUNDATIONS OF
AROMA FREEDOM

Chapter 1

My Journey to Aroma Freedom and Beyond

I wrote my first book, "The Aroma Freedom Technique" in 2016. That book was the culmination of 20 years of clinical psychotherapy practice, research, and experimentation with many traditional and non-traditional psychotherapy and healing methods, along with 15 years of experience using essential oils.

Prior to writing that book, I had developed a method for using essential oils to dissolve and transform traumatic memories. It had shown itself to be extremely gentle, fast, and effective for clients struggling with traumatic and troubling memories.

In fact, it was so successful, I had been invited to do a tour of Japan, Singapore, Malaysia and Hong Kong to demonstrate this technique to people who already used essential oils but needed to know the specifics of how they worked for trauma.

On trips like this, I always had terrible jet lag. My body just did not adjust quickly to the time changes, and I would regularly find myself up in the middle of the night, unable to sleep, in a hotel lobby by myself. Because sleep was out of the question, I decided to start writing some notes about a book I wanted to write. I did not yet know what the book would be about exactly but figured that it would emerge as I scribbled my thoughts.

The driving question I had at that time was this: I knew that the technique I created worked well for the "big T" traumas such as car accidents, assaults, abuse, etc....but what about all the "little t" traumas that people experienced every day, such as the hurts, disappointments, frustrations of everyday life?

Could there be a technique that would work for those types of problems?

In my daily walks through bookstores, I came across a book called "The Trauma of Everyday Life." I bought it, thinking that this was exactly what I was going to be writing about. To my horror, the book was not about resolving those traumas, but just living with them. The basic message of the book was basically "Hey, everyday life is traumatic. Deal with it."

I knew that this was not the message I wanted to give, nor the direction I wanted to go.

I put into words the things that I had noticed during my years of practicing psychotherapy and essential oil use, such as:

- When people set goals, they usually get a barrage of negative thoughts telling them why they cannot accomplish them.

- These thoughts usually lead to negative feelings, such as

sadness, frustration, or anger.

- When a feeling is named, it starts to lose its power to scare us, and reveal what the solution might be.

- When a strong feeling or emotion surfaces, it tends to rise and then fall like a wave, if the person is just able to stay present and feel the feeling without running away from it, distracting themselves, or judging it as good or bad.

- All feelings have a bodily component, and noticing the bodily reaction helps the feeling to emerge more clearly.

- Feelings trigger memories of other times we felt the same way.

- Early events in our lives tend to leave "memory complexes" that can interfere with daily functioning.

- Smelling certain essential oils seems to be balancing and calming to people - but I did not yet know how to integrate them into my clinical practice, other than to resolve traumatic memories.

At that time, I was reading a fabulous book, called "The Untethered Soul" by Michael Singer. In that book, Singer discussed what he called the "Inner Roommate." This is the inner voice that is always with you and who gives a running commentary to every thought you have and action you perform. It is the voice that is constantly commenting, questioning, doubting, arguing, and interpreting life in each moment.

Singer shared how he learned to meditate and to just notice the inner voice rather than react or respond to it, and in this way was able to find a kind of freedom that was exhilarating and deeply peaceful at the same time.

Reading this sparked an idea within me: rather than just noticing the voice in a state of passive awareness (witness consciousness), what if we pay attention to the _feeling_ that the voice evokes? What if, when we think about our dreams and goals, and the inner roommate tells us we cannot accomplish them, we notice how that feels? Where do we feel it in the body? What memory does that trigger?

In this way, we arrive back at memories where _something_ happened. It may be a traumatic memory, but it might also just be a relatively trivial incident, something that you hadn't thought about in years. I realized that perhaps this was the kind of "non-traumatic" incident that we could clear with essential oils.

Armed with this fresh inspiration, I returned home from my trip to Asia and announced to my family that I was ready to write the book I had been wanting to write for so long. I gave myself 30 days to write it, because there was going to be a convention I wanted to present it at in 60 days and I figured that would give me enough time to also get it printed and delivered (I had never done that before, it was just a guess).

Every day I went to the library to write, and in the beginning, I was just organizing my ideas, taking notes, finding interesting articles and books related to my topic, etc. As I pulled the ideas together, I had the inspiration to create a step-by-step process that would take a person all the way from thinking of a goal or intention, through identifying and clearing out the negative thoughts, feelings, and memories that emerged, to finally arriving at an affirmation and action step to make the goal a reality.

With this, the 12 Step Aroma Freedom Technique was born. I tested the technique on myself and noticed how well it worked, and that I was able to make any negative thoughts about my goals simply dissolve. I took it home and tested it on my wife, Elaine, and daughter, Eyana, and the same thing happened. I knew I was onto something! Through further testing with clients, friends, and anyone I could find, I became convinced that this process worked in a way that was repeatable and could be done by anyone.

All this was wonderful, but it was also the case that I was down to just 15 days left (out of my original 30) to accomplish my goal of writing my book in time to have it at the convention. I did not have much time…but I did have the new technique. So, I tested it on myself once again. I knew that setting this goal would trigger all of my doubts that it could happen.

Here is a rough transcript of what happened next:

Me: "I am going to write my book within 15 days."

Inner voice: "That's impossible, that is too much pressure, nobody can do that"

Negative feelings: sadness, discouragement, hopelessness, anger

Bodily sensations: tight belly, eyes downcast

Memories that surfaced: To be honest, I don't remember what memories surfaced.

Essential Oils: Frankincense, Lavender, Stress Away Blend (see appendix)

I breathed the oils into the memories, and the memories dissolved, the negative voices went away, and my bodily sensations relaxed.

A new thought emerged - "No problem. A 150 page book is just 10 pages a day for 15 days. How hard is that?"

I was filled with a newfound energy and excitement. I knew it could happen. That it _would_ happen.

I created an affirmation and put it on my refrigerator: "I write 10 pages of my book today."

Every day, I said my affirmation before going to the library.

For the first several days of writing, I addressed the big topics I wanted to cover, such as the power of the sense of smell, how essential oils work, how we get stuck emotionally, and the nature of traumatic memories and how they are stored differently in the brain than less emotionally charged memories.

It was only after several days that it became clear to me the book was actually going to be about the 12 step technique itself. Once that became obvious, I knew exactly what I needed to say in order to finish the book on time, and I was even more motivated, excited, and confident that it would be done on time.

Sure enough, on day 15, I told my wife that I had completed the book. Now we just had to find a title, cover, foreword, endorsements, ISBN number, printer, online store, etc.

I quickly realized that climbing to the top of one mountain just means there is a valley below to traverse on the way to the next peak, and that the journey was just beginning! This is when I really had to put The Aroma Freedom Technique to the test.

For each problem that we had to solve, I simply set a new goal - such as finding the right title, getting the cover to look how we wanted, navigating websites and printers, etc. - and then I did The Aroma Freedom Technique (AFT for short) on myself to clear away any doubt that the goal could be accomplished.

For instance, my wife, Elaine, and I had discussions like the following:

Me: "Here is a book cover I put together - what do you think?"

Elaine: "The title is OK, but the book is ugly. Can you try again?"

Me: "OK, how about this one?"

Elaine: "I don't like the colors."

Me: "Does it really matter what the colors are? We have to get this to the printer or it won't be ready in time for the convention! We don't have time to fiddle with the colors."

Elaine: "I'm sorry, but I can't support a book that is not beautiful."

Me: I felt the frustration rising in my chest. Doesn't she realize we don't have time to make it beautiful? I took this as a cue to breathe some essential oils into the feelings - probably the Stress-Away Blend - and after a minute the sense of pressure dissolved and was replaced by a renewed feeling of hope and patience about the process. Then I said, "I will go back to the drawing board."

In that way, we were able to meet our very tight deadline and arrive at the convention the same day as the books arrived there from the printer!

In the first book I told the story, worth repeating here, about how my brain shut down during the very fast (3 day) editing phase I was doing before publishing the book.

I had been working with my friend on the final run-through of the entire book, going over each paragraph to make sure it said what I intended it to say. On the second day, I told her that my brain had stopped working. I just could no longer think clearly.

I decided to take a walk to clear my head, and I brought my essential oils with me. Realizing that perhaps there was an emotional issue being triggered, I took myself through an AFT session. In that session, I set a goal to finish the editing and get the book to the printer.

Then, I identified the related negative thoughts and feelings, and found myself back at a memory of a time in high school when I had lost a track race.

As I breathed the oils into the memory (later you will learn more about what that actually means), I caught hold of a specific negative thought that was emerging. I heard a voice in my head say, **"You're not strong enough to finish."**

In that moment, it became clear that losing the track race had triggered a negative thought process that had been sitting in my subconscious mind for 30 years. I had not thought about that memory since it happened many years ago, as it was not particularly traumatic to me.

However, the process of _sprinting_ to finish the editing had clearly triggered similar feelings to what I had in high school when I was sprinting in the 1 mile race and ran out of steam and could not finish strong.

Once this became clear and I continued to breathe the oils into the memory, the whole scene faded, the negative thoughts and feelings vanished, and most importantly, my brain turned back on!

I confidently walked back to my house, told my friend I was ready, and we finished the editing process.

I share this story to highlight a couple of things:

1. Negative experiences do not need to be particularly

traumatic to have a deep and long lasting influence on us.

2. A negative, subconscious thought/voice can lay dormant for decades, only to resurface at exactly the point when you want to do something that challenges the perspective it holds.

3. Using a process like AFT (Aroma Freedom Technique) to overcome challenges can be the difference between finishing a task and almost finishing a task (which, in the case of a book or project, is the difference between it happening and it not happening).

The events that followed my printing and sharing the book at the convention are a blur, because they happened so fast. Briefly:

Many people expressed interest in the book and purchased it. One in particular said she wanted me to do a zoom call with her team to take them all through the AFT process. I had never done a zoom call before (this was 2016), and I did not know how it would work to lead an online group. Nevertheless, we did the call and people were blown away at the changes they noticed in their emotional state. Several of them asked me "Can I get certified in this?"

I had not considered certification, so I just said, "Sure, maybe in a couple of years."

A few days later, I led a group in Singapore through the same process via zoom. Again, people were amazed. Again, they asked about certification. Again, I told them "Maybe in a couple of years."

That night, I was lying awake in bed thinking about what was happening. People were asking me for a certification. I didn't know where to start with that request. Then, I remembered how, every time I felt blocked, the AFT process would show me the next step.

So, I went downstairs to my office (I worked from home), and did a session on myself. I set a goal of creating an AFT Certification. As soon as I did this, sure enough, the negative voices appeared:

"You don't know how to do that"

"How would you assess competence?"

"What will you teach them?"

"How long will it last?"

"How much will you charge?"

I just followed the AFT steps and identified the feelings, bodily sensations, and memories that were triggered. I put essential oils on my hands and breathed them into the memories. The memories and feelings faded.

Then, just as before, a new awareness came into me. I "downloaded" a course outline very quickly and easily. I realized that it should be an 8 week course on zoom, with topics from the book, lots of practice sessions, etc.

Since I was managing my own website at that time, I just put the course announcement on the website, sent a quick email out about the course, and went back to bed.

To my surprise, by morning when I looked at my email, 5 people from Singapore had already registered for Certification! I knew at that point that there was something really big happening. I emailed my registrants that I could start in September (it was July, less than a month after publishing the book). They said, "Why can't you start now?" I agreed, and sure enough a week later the first certification was launched.

Two months later, we launched the second certification group. By this point I realized that I was helping more people by teaching them Aroma Freedom than I had ever been able to help seeing clients 1-1 in my office. I officially closed my office that I had been in for 20 years, and I have been teaching Aroma Freedom full-time since then.

Over the last 6 years, I have had the privilege to teach and mentor hundreds of students as they became Certified Aroma Freedom Practitioners. I have seen people transformed from shy, depressed, or under-achieving people with passion but no platform, into confident, purpose-filled practitioners helping people with these techniques and loving it. Along the way, we have also been able to refine The Aroma Freedom Technique and go from 1 Master Technique (AFT) to 6 Aroma Freedom Techniques to cover past, present, and future. We also have learned so much about the neuroscience of why it works, how to tweak it to work even better for more people, and how it fits into other therapies or coaching approaches. And we are still learning.

My life looks radically different now than it did before I discovered Aroma Freedom, and how I help people is different as well.

Before Aroma Freedom, I saw clients in my office individually, or as a couple, and I used whatever skills I had developed by then to help them. If I didn't know the answer, I would read a book, talk to a colleague, or take training to improve my services. I enjoyed this, and my clients generally benefited.

However, there were some problems with this way of working:

1. I could only help 1-2 people at a time. This meant 6-8 per day, or about 25 per week on an average week.

2. It was tiring for me. It kept me sitting for hours, and sometimes I would feel drained by the end of the day.

3. My clients made progress, but sometimes very slowly.

4. Even when clients felt better, they were not empowered to help anyone else. The skills that I had used in helping them were not transferred to them in the process. This kept me very busy (always new referrals), but I imagine there were thousands of people who needed help and didn't get it.

After Aroma Freedom, it is a much different picture:

1. I help dozens (sometimes hundreds!) of people at once

through online courses and training.

2. It is energizing for me to see so many people having powerful transformations every day. Working online, I can choose where to teach from, whether to stand or sit, and when I want to work. In fact, my family and I have traveled extensively in the last 8 years. I can start and stop my work now, according to my wishes and inspirations.

3. Clients now make amazing shifts in every session. They also don't need me as much. Once they have made the shift they need, they go and live their life and come back when they need a tune-up. Or, they take part in a larger course, such as Practitioner Certification, or perhaps one on self-love, grief, business, etc. and use these sessions to become more empowered and successful.

4. Perhaps most importantly, my clients and students learn the techniques and can go out and help themselves, family, friends, and even their own clients. They collectively impact thousands more people than I ever could by myself. And, they are empowered to help themselves in a way that would have been unimaginable for my clients before.

The purpose of this book is to show you the Aroma Freedom processes so that you can discover for yourself how easy it can be to help yourself and others move past obstacles, get unstuck, and live a life full of meaning and purpose. Some of the techniques just take a minute or two, others will take a little longer as you identify and clear out deeply embedded memories that have been influencing your life in ways you don't yet fully understand.

Key Chapter Takeaways

Aroma Freedom is a synthesis of over 20 years of both clinical and academic research, practice, and integration of psychology and aromatherapy.

Aroma Freedom was born from a desire to find a faster and gentler solution to the problem of negative thoughts, feelings and memories.

The practice is deeply personal, and I have used the Aroma Freedom protocols to further my own personal and professional development every step of the way.

Aroma Freedom has replaced most of what I used to do as a psychologist because it is so effective and integrates other approaches I used to use.

Chapter 2

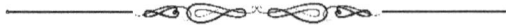

How Aroma Freedom changes lives

In the last chapter, I shared the personal and professional transformation that I have experienced since discovering Aroma Freedom. In this chapter, I will share some stories from students, Aroma Freedom Practitioners, and clients to illustrate exactly how Aroma Freedom has impacted them.

But first, let's talk about the kind of freedom that Aroma Freedom can bring.

There are many kinds of freedom, just as there are many kinds of bondage.

Freedom of Expression

The freedom to express oneself openly has been argued to be a fundamental human right. But before it is even a political question, it is a psychological question. You can ask yourself:

"Do I feel free to say what I think, feel and believe, or do I have something within me that's stopping me from doing that? Am I censoring my own thoughts?"

When you feel free to express yourself, you feel comfortable talking to people, presenting your knowledge and ideas to them, asking for what you want and need, in short, being seen by them. This inner freedom of expression translates into the outer freedom of being able to succeed in relationships, in business, and in your life as a whole.

When you are too concerned about not making mistakes, being perfect, or making a good impression, you are unable to be yourself authentically with others.

One of the primary benefits people experience with Aroma Freedom is the inner freedom to show the world who they are in a comfortable and confident way.

Anne was a student in our Practitioner Certification Program. When she first came into class, she was very nervous about the prospect of showing up online and speaking to people. During the training program, I have the students do a lot of sessions on themselves to clear out their fears of showing up and being successful. We helped Anne to process and transform several memories that had been interfering with her ability to be comfortable online. After the program, the changes she noticed were very palpable:

Anne Stark Hummeldorf I can now do FB Lives and online Webinars and before I was completely uncomfortable and tongue-tied. Thank you Dr. Benjamin Perkus!

Like · Reply · 1w   2

The fear of public speaking has been said to be even more

prevalent than the fear of death! When people are afraid of showing up in front of people, either in-person or online, it is likely because as children they encountered some negative messages connected with expressing themselves. Or, their personality was just more private and self-controlled. In any case, this fear of "appearing" can have detrimental effects on life in both personal and professional realms. On the other hand, when the freedom of expression is restored, there is a wonderful calm and peace that can be felt.

Stacey is a coach and Aroma Freedom Practitioner who used to be afraid to market her practice. After using Aroma Freedom to rid herself of these fears, she is now able to talk to prospective clients and feel much more comfortable:

> Stacey Ross I find the "no" from clients and prospects no longer affects me! I approach them with confidence in knowing I'll be okay if they say no to what I'm offering or they can say yes, and either way I'll be ok!!
>
> Like · Reply · 1w

Many times, the fear of expressing oneself can hinder business success. Especially if you are in sales or are an entrepreneur, you need to feel comfortable talking to people about who you are, what you do, and what you charge. By conquering the fear of rejection, Stacey was able to feel much more confident in her business and in her life.

If you struggle with freedom of expression, you will benefit from The Aroma Freedom Technique (AFT) described in Chapter 8. You can set a goal related to expressing yourself confidently and comfortably, and then watch and see what hidden memories and thoughts surface that have been holding you back. Using essential oils in the way that I describe will allow those memories to quickly be transformed and you will begin to see your confidence rise in social situations.

Freedom from Negative Moods, Behaviors, or Habits

Can you choose how you want to feel in a particular situation? Can you act in alignment with who you want to be, or do you feel driven by cravings, compulsions, and self-destructive habits?

If you're in a bad mood, it colors the whole day. The sun might be shining. There might be nice things happening. But if you're in a sour mood, you can't really enjoy it. You might then turn to addictive substances, distractions, or negative behaviors instead of coping productively with what is happening in your life.

One way of describing inner freedom is the ability to feel peace and pleasant feelings even in the midst of stress, challenges, hurts, or disappointment. In other words, the ability not to let negative external events ruin your inner landscape.

Aroma Freedom teaches you how to "ride the wave" of feelings that come throughout a day, and not get stuck in the negative ones. It also clears out the deep, hidden causes of negative moods and feelings, so that you no longer need to fight with yourself just to maintain a positive outlook.

Jennifer overcame many years of using food to manage her emotions when she realized how to process and release the negative emotions with Aroma Freedom. Now she is a Certified Practitioner who helps women daily with the same issues she used to have.

Jennifer Zazula Miskiel I feel in control of my emotions. I am not scared anymore that I will be overpowered by them.

Like · Reply · 1w

Kayla is a practitioner who used to have several anxious habits, such as hair pulling and nail biting. Since learning and using Aroma Freedom, these habits are a thing of the past. Even more important is the fact that she no longer gets as upset in difficult situations:

Kayla Marie Schnider I pulled my hair as a calming thing with my anxiety. After awhile, it became a habit. After AFT, I don't pull my hair. I don't tend to get as worked up or overwhelmed in difficult situations either. I have also been a nail bighter my whole life. One AFT session, and I have long nails! I even made it through Super Bowl with my nails being a Chiefs fan 😌 🏈

Like · Reply · 1w · Edited

○ 2

These changes did not occur by fighting with the habits using "willpower" or "accountability." Rather, they occurred as the natural byproduct of processing unresolved thoughts, feelings and memories, and learning how to address feelings as they come up in a natural and spontaneous way.

Erika used to be triggered easily into rage, anger, and irritation. She was not in control of how she felt, and was at the mercy of people and situations in her life.

Erika Vaughn Bartlett Just one?! Everything use to trigger me into a rage or extreme irritation. Now it rolls of my shoulders. My whole life has changed. I am forever thankful for the gift you gave me Benjamin Perkus. Didn't know I could ever be "normal"

Like · Reply · 1w

Being triggered by everyday events is usually a symptom of unresolved prior life experiences, whether recent or from childhood. Often, however, the person has no idea that this is occurring. They respond to each new event as a catastrophe, rather than being able to just tackle it for the small, manageable event that it usually is.

If you find yourself emotionally triggered by minor irritations, or that you are leaning on addictive substances such as sugar, alcohol, tobacco, etc., you will benefit from the Aroma Clear Technique (Chapter 14). This process helps to very quickly identify specific unresolved memories that are being triggered by everyday situations. It can be used at any time when stress is causing you to behave in a way that you don't like. You will also benefit from the Aroma Freedom Cravings Protocol (see how to access bonus content at the end of this book for a link).

This brings us to one of the most important kinds of freedom that people need, and which Aroma Freedom provides abundantly, which is:

Freedom from Painful Memories

We all have had tragedies in our lives. Some people have been blessed with relatively few painful events in their lives, had a happy childhood, a successful family and career, and a life full of meaning and purpose. Most people, however, have had their share of hurts, disappointments, or even trauma, abuse, and intense loss.

When traumatic events occur, they leave an indelible mark on a person. They affect personality development when they occur in younger years. Trauma in childhood or adulthood can lead to PTSD (Post Traumatic Stress Disorder), depression, anxiety, and a host of other physical and emotional problems.

Unlike traditional "talk therapy," Aroma Freedom offers a fast, gentle, and effective way to become free of these negative events permanently and without side effects.

Marije was able to release a very painful memory from when her father passed away. She can now think of the event without becoming upset at all:

> Marije Wagenmakers I can now think about the time my dad died without getting choked up and being right back in that moment (I was 11).... I still can't believe that all that emotional charge is gone after carrying it for 30 years! 💕
>
> Like · Reply · 1w   1

Time is no barrier to the effectiveness of Aroma Freedom. Even events that occurred decades ago can be quickly processed and released. Before using Aroma Freedom, she was haunted by the memory, and now there is simply not an emotional charge when thinking about it. This, of course, allows her to devote her emotional energy to her current life, as well as giving her the ability to pursue her goals and dreams for the future.

Anneloes found Aroma Freedom to be more powerful than EMDR (Eye Movement Desensitization and Reprocessing, a trauma processing technique commonly used in psychotherapy) in releasing negative feelings and emotions related to past, traumatic events:

> **Anneloes Mulder** It has helped me tremendously with dealing with my PTSD. I had EMDR before, but that did not solve nearly as much as AFT did. Now I can leave all the negative feelings and emotions attached to the events that caused my PTSD behind me and live a brighte... See More
>
> Like · Reply · 1w
>
> 2

As she says, she is able to "leave it all behind" so she can move forward.

Jenny was able to let go of old hurts and beliefs from childhood:

> **Jenny Mehler** AFT has helped me process and release old hurts and beliefs that I've been carrying around since childhood. It's become my go-to tool for dealing with worry and anxiousness - AFT leaves me with a feeling of peace, lightness, and a new insight into what was troubling with me.
>
> Like · Reply · 1w · Edited
>
> 4

By letting go of the past, she is able to feel peace and lightness. She also gains insight and awareness about what the real problems and solutions are for her.

Brenda had been struggling with memories that she had been previously unaware of surfacing into her mind. This caused her extreme distress until she used Aroma Freedom to dissolve and resolve the memories:

> **Brenda Marie** Repressed memories. They started to come out a few years ago and I then was in a state of panic. AFT helped process them and disconnect the intensity of them. I cannot imagine my life without AFT. Freedom and peace now!
>
> Like · Reply · 1w

> Being haunted by upsetting memories is one of the most painful experiences you can have, and can leave you feeling powerless, hopeless, and disconnected from others. Chapter 7 (The Miracle of Memory Reconsolidation) explains the science behind how Aroma Freedom helps to change these memories forever. Then, Chapter 9 (TMRT) describes the exact procedure you can use to process and resolve these memories in a gentle and yet profound way.

Freedom from Powerlessness and Victimization

Joni was able to overcome many physical and emotional health issues that had been caused by prior victimization. By using Aroma Freedom she was able to become a survivor instead of a victim:

> Joni Gorman Conlon severe anxiety/chronic health issues due to a life of abuse (as a child and I married an abuser) AFT has been the most effective tool in allowing me to move through "all the stuff" that comes with that. I AM Living the Life of a SURVIVOR rather than a VICTIM. Peace! 🖤
>
> Like · Reply · 1w

Kim was able to work through issues of forgiveness and healing from betrayal, and she noticed a palpable, physical release as the Aroma Freedom process worked within her. Whenever we have physical problems, it is impossible to know how much of this comes from "physical" causes, and how much comes from "emotional" causes. In these cases, I always encourage people to "give it a try." When the emotional baggage has been lifted, we are in a better position to see how much physical pain is "leftover." It may be that the physical distress completely disappears. Or, it may be that there is still physical distress. In that case, you will be in a better position to know what to do to heal the physical condition once you are in a better space emotionally.

> **Kim McBride Feldbaum** Forgiveness 💜
> I had been stuck for a decade with the lingering hurt and the anger of a family members' betrayal.
> AFT supported me in identifying where in my body I was holding onto the feelings and allowed me to release and heal my heart and gut spaces. 💜 🩸 🤍
> I feel lighter as if a tremendous weight has been lifted both physically and emotionally. 🙏 🤍
> I am grateful for AFT supporting me forgiving my family member 🤍
>
> Like · Reply · 1w

Christine is another practitioner whose healing was related to releasing shame and guilt surrounding a trauma that occurred when she was a teenager. She had been carrying this around for decades and it had affected her marriage as well as her relationship with herself. Once she released the emotional attachment to those memories, she was able to embrace feelings of self-love and self-worth, and inner strength:

> **Christine Nardone Riccardi** Self Love... I Am Beautiful I Am Strong I Am Worthy 🤍 Thank you for helping make my life more beautiful 🤍
>
> Like · Reply · 1w   👍 4

Moving from feelings of victimization and powerlessness to ones of self-acceptance and empowerment is a common factor when you begin to use all of the Aroma Freedom Techniques to resolve old hurts, negative memories, and negative beliefs. In Chapter 10, I describe some specific mindset shifts that will help you to understand and embrace a "growth mindset" and claim the "Spirit of Freedom" that is your birthright. This is possible whether you use these processes on yourself, or if you seek out a certified practitioner to help you through them.

Freedom from Paralysis and Self-Doubt

Nothing is more frustrating than knowing what you want to do, but feeling paralyzed and unable to act in the direction of your goals and dreams. Yet this is a very common problem. When you have self-doubt, you tend to "overthink" your actions, and then you can "talk yourself out of" doing the very things you need to do.

The problem of procrastination has deep psychological roots and we will be exploring those in Chapter 12 when describing the Aroma Boost Technique. It is common for people who start using Aroma Freedom to notice that suddenly they are getting more things done, projects left abandoned years ago are being finished, and toxic or inappropriate relationships are being fixed or left behind.

Amanda went from feelings of paralysis and inability to act, to being able to move forward and have more healthy, appropriate relationships:

> Amanda Horne Buckner I used to feel crushed and paralyzed by some certain circumstances. Now I'm able to move forward. AFT has also allowed me to put healthy boundaries in place. It has truly been life changing for me.
>
> Like · Reply · 1w · Edited

The Aroma Boost Technique (Chapter 12) tackles procrastination by dissolving its two main roots: Task Aversiveness, and Future Time Discounting. In the Aroma Boost, you will learn how to enjoy tasks that you have been dreading, and to experience heightened levels of motivation for acting right away instead of putting things off into the indefinite future.

Freedom of Self-Forgiveness + Inner Guidance

We have all made mistakes, and have done things that we later regretted. Sometimes these were actions we took, and sometimes these were actions we neglected to take. When we judge ourselves harshly, it dampens our ability to live in the present and to pursue future goals. And yet, our past mistakes also serve as a reminder of what **not** to do and who we **don't** want to be. They are important guideposts in our journey to being a person we can respect and who can be looked up to by others. How can we integrate past experiences in a way that both teaches us the lesson we needed to learn, while still allowing us to move forward?

Resolving past experiences is a critical part of what happens during Memory Reconsolidation (Chapter 7). The goal of Aroma Freedom is not so much to just "release" painful memories, but rather, to integrate the memories and what happened in a way that allows us to learn any lessons that those experiences had to offer. By doing this, the memories lose their emotional charge and no longer hinder our progress in life.

Anita was able to find self-forgiveness for a decision she had made years ago. She now has a better understanding of the situation and her role in it:

Anita Grosso I didn't know that it was possible to find Self-forgiveness for a poor decision made many years ago. The clarity I got, through the process, opened up my reasoning in a different way for better understanding of the events that led to the decision

Like · Reply · 1w

Gaining the ability to glean the wisdom that experiences have to offer, and to have access to your own inner guidance and intuition, is an important part of the changes that occur when you begin to use Aroma Freedom. In addition to resolving past experiences, you need to be able to look at upcoming future events, decisions, and choices, and to feel a sense of guidance or comfort in knowing you are going in the right direction.

The Aroma Wisdom Technique (Chapter 13) provides a pathway for moving from worry and dread, to a sense of wisdom and guidance in the face of an unknown and unknowable future.

Freedom to Help Others

When you begin to taste the freedom that comes from releasing old unwanted patterns of thought and behavior, there is a natural progression towards wanting to help others become free as well. After all, what is the fun of becoming free yourself, when everyone around you is still in bondage to their old patterns?

Aroma Freedom gives everyone the opportunity not just to help themselves, but to help others as well. In fact, this was one of the driving forces behind the creation of techniques in the first place. For many years I had been researching new ways to help people in my Clinical Psychology practice. I would regularly attend new conferences and trainings, and then come back to try what I had learned on my clients. Alongside my clinical practice, my wife and I had learned about Essential Oils and would hold weekend workshops and classes to teach people how to use them for their personal wellness.

One of the principles that went with teaching people how to use the oils for wellness is that what we taught needed to be "duplicatable." In other words, if they had to come back to us over and over for us to teach them and their friends, then they weren't truly empowered to stand on their own. As much as possible, we taught them using books, videos, and presentations that they could also go and teach others with - thus, in a sense, "duplicating" our teachings.

On the other hand, as I mentioned in my story in Chapter One, I was only able to help one person at a time in my Psychology practice. And, when they went home, none of what I did to help them was "duplicatable" - meaning, they could not turn around and help anyone in their life in the way that I had helped them.

After many years of leading this "double life" (of being a Psychologist by day and an essential oils educator on the side), I was at a crossroads. I felt that both sides of my career and life were important, and I didn't want to give up either one.

In 2015, I spoke to one of my mentors. I explained my predicament, of how I did not want to give up either side but did not see how to integrate them. She thought about this for a moment, and then said: "Create a tool. This will allow others to do what you do."

With that comment, a light bulb went off in my head. If I could find a way to create a **system** of using the oils to help people psychologically, and put it in a format that others could use and follow, then I would have accomplished the feat of "duplication," but this time in the psychological realm. I could then not only teach others how to help themselves outside of my clinical office, but they could then turn around and help others using the system.

This is exactly what we now have with the various Aroma Freedom techniques. It has allowed thousands of people to learn to use the processes on themselves, and then on others.

In our training program, students are asked to work on themselves as much as they work on others. Additionally, the very task of becoming masterful at this technique will trigger many of the emotional issues that have been holding the students back from being as effective as they could be.

Mary is a therapist/healer in Australia who worked through some powerful memories during her training to become a certified practitioner. She had become aware of a fear that would surface within her while working with clients. This was obviously distressing, and yet she did not have any conscious understanding of where the fear was coming from. Through the course of the training we facilitated several clearings of early childhood memories that allowed her to move completely beyond these fears:

Mary Girishaa An unexplained fear that would surface as I began working with a client, a feeling that it wasn't safe to do this work. This expressed as a physical tremor in my hands making it difficult, embarrassing to do my hands on treatments. AF has helped me understand the memories and clear the emotional charge so I can do my work...to feel safe. 🙏🙏🙏

Like · Reply · 1w

Students in the program regularly tell me that the personal growth they experience during training was at least as valuable as learning how to use the techniques professionally. Plus, they say that the feeling they get when helping people find freedom using these techniques is incomparable - to see someone go from feelings of hopelessness and despair to hope and excitement in less than an hour is absolutely exhilarating!

To learn more about the training programs we offer for both professionals and laypeople, see Chapters 15 and 16.

Some data on the effectiveness of AFT:

Here are the results of some research we did on the effectiveness of AFT for boosting personal confidence. When I first ran the certification course back in 2016, I had each student record all of their practice sessions in a google form. I asked them to be very specific, recording each goal, thought, feeling, and rating from 0-10. We did this for about a year, and when I went back to look at the data, I found that Google had organized this data very nicely. This is data from over 3400 client sessions.

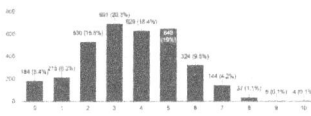

INITIAL INTENTION RATING
HOW POSSIBLE DOES IT FEEL?
3,411 RESPONSES

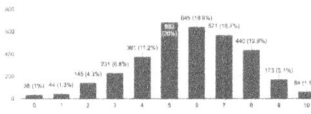

AFTER ONE ROUND
HOW POSSIBLE DOES IT FEEL NOW?
3,411 RESPONSES

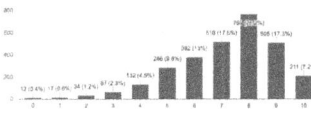

AFTER TWO ROUNDS
HOW POSSIBLE DOES IT FEEL NOW?
2,938 RESPONSES

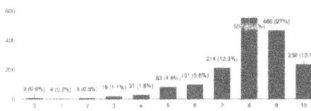

AFTER THREE ROUNDS
HOW POSSIBLE DOES IT FEEL NOW?
1,733 RESPONSES

The results show that the effect of Aroma Freedom was consistent across thousands of client sessions, with those sessions being performed by hundreds of practitioners. This is significant because it means both that:

A. The results people got with Aroma Freedom were consistent across clients. Over the course of 3400 sessions, the trends from low levels of confidence to high levels of confidence about reaching goals did not vary. This means we are tapping into a core process that works for a wide variety of people.

B. The results were consistent across a large number of practitioners. This means that the results came from the teachable, duplicatable, step-by-step process of Aroma Freedom, and not from the skills and training of a single practitioner or creator such as myself. It means that anyone who follows these steps can be successful.

From the graphs, you can see that the client's initial rating was, on average, in the 3-5 range (relatively hopeless about reaching the goal). After one round, the average rating was in the 5-6 range. After two rounds, it was about an 8 average rating. And after 3 rounds (this is as far as we tracked), it was clearly 8++. Clients moved from hopeless to confident in about 30-45 minutes, over and over.

Case Study: Janell Rardon - Psychotherapist

Janell is a psychotherapist in Virginia who was invited to learn about Aroma Freedom shortly after finishing her first book. As it turned out, her book publishing got delayed for reasons beyond her control, and in the interim what she learned through Aroma Freedom was so powerful, she decided to alter the book to include some references to Aroma Freedom. Here is what she said:

"A friend invited me to attend an event that introduced me to a new and revolutionary emotional health modality, Aroma Freedom Technique, developed by clinical psychologist Dr. Benjamin Perkus.... This simple, safe, and highly efficient healing modality incorporates several different psychological therapies, including EMDR (eye movement desensitization and reprocessing), with the power of aromatherapy and the use of memory reconsolidation—the brain's natural way of updating and learning.

Through the years, I have had many clients who remained stuck in unhealthy behavior patterns. They kept tripping over the same root, no matter how hard we worked to dig it out. We couldn't resolve the mystery, and I committed to staying the course until we did.

In my personal story, my mother's harsh prosody, or tone of voice, activated a memory or memories that still had a five-alarm negative charge attached to it. Even with all the counseling and therapy I have done, that specific tone of voice still activated me. It triggered something deep in my subconscious and instantly upset me. As I've come to learn, the harsh sound of her tone of voice toward my sister was something that made me feel unsafe and insecure—as a child. Those memories were stored deep in my implicit memory system…until I used Aroma Freedom to clear them out.

Following certification, when I started using Aroma Freedom with clients, I saw a credible difference in my work with my clients, particularly my trauma-informed clients. As I carefully guided clients through the twelve steps of the Aroma Freedom Technique, they breathed strategically formulated essential oils that immediately activated memory reconsolidation, removing any negative energy and obstacles, and gently began creating new, healthy neural pathways."

Case Study: Penelope Layzell - Corporate Trainer and Coach

"I came across Aroma Freedom back in the summer last year, and it immediately excited me as I had just become a certified 5th dimension earth healer and upon trying out the practice myself immediately saw the benefits for stress and anxiety reduction, as well as an increase in productivity.

It was upon searching for the process after the challenge that I came across the practitioner course and immediately knew I needed to undertake this so that as I transitioned from the corporate world into that of a Spiritual Life Coach that this would be a huge part of what I did.

I can't tell you how strongly this process has impacted my world personally. I work in a very target driven stressful environment and know how to manage and avoid stress and burnout, (it is these techniques I have been called to bring to the world) and I started using the process in my life daily and noticed how incredible the shifts were.

An example of this was I needed to revisit the charge rates for all clients, a massive undertaking, and I was expected to achieve it within a short period of time. Figures and math are not my strong points. I was the last manager to begin the course, but this occurred at the time I was practicing the Aroma Boost on myself as part of the course. Not only did I get through the review but I finished ahead of the other managers! This was pivotal to me really becoming excited about the potential of working with clients using this process.

I carry my oils around with me everywhere now, and at any moment will undertake an Aroma Reset when stressful situations arise.

Seeing the shifts in others has only cemented the belief that this process is life changing. I have witnessed people literally evolve in front of me from inward focus to becoming so self assured.

Having lived in perpetual burnout until a life changing illness turned my life around 6 years ago, I self taught myself healing techniques to connect back to myself and understand and manage stress. I stopped having debilitating panic attacks and navigating anxiety and this led to me becoming a certified healer. I have a big vision of changing the way the 9-5 corporate world works and have started transitioning into setting up my own coaching business to help lead clients to successful fulfilled lives without the stress and burnout. These oils will be an essential part of the programs and training that I will offer to my clients. In fact once I saw how incredible these oils are, I put a hold on launching my business because I didn't want to launch without having this tool available for clients!

Key Chapter Takeaways

Aroma Freedom has been used to develop many kinds of freedom, including:

- Freedom of expression
- Freedom from negative moods, behaviors, or habits
- Freedom from painful memories
- Freedom from powerlessness and victimization
- Freedom from paralysis and self-doubt
- Freedom of self-forgiveness and inner guidance
- Freedom to help others

Outcome research shows a reliable and consistent improvement in confidence that one's goals can be reached.

Aroma Freedom can help therapists and coaches to be even more effective.

AROMA FREEDOM

Chapter 3

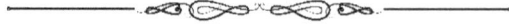

Personal and Professional
Freedom

As I mentioned in Chapter 1, creating Aroma Freedom radically changed my life, both personally and professionally. And it can change yours, too, if you choose to take the journey.

If you are a person who desires to become free in some of the ways I discussed in the last chapter, then this book is for you. You don't have to be a mental health professional to use these simple processes for greater individual freedom. That being said, if you are a psychotherapist, coach, or healing arts professional, Aroma Freedom represents a revolution in how your practice will look and the scope and pace of the results you can get for your clients.

From a personal perspective, all human beings suffer under similar limitations. We are all born into a particular family and culture, and as we grow, our experiences shape the structure of how we perceive the world and ourselves. We reach adulthood with specific beliefs about who we are, what we are capable of, and what we are NOT capable of. Becoming free of such conditioning is the first stage in finding and then expressing your authentic self.

Professional therapists and coaches, similarly, are also bound by the limits of the training and experience they have had. They were taught specific models of healing that correspond to whichever theoretical orientation they subscribe to. The model of therapy or coaching that a practitioner uses will help some of their clients more than others. Yet most practitioners, if they truly want to help their clients, will desire to always improve their craft and find a better way - something that is more effective, more empowering, more predictably helpful, and frankly, easier to do, day-in and day-out.

As you read through this chapter and the rest of the book, I highly recommend you take the time to complete the assessments you find there. This will allow you to see, from within your own experience, both where you may be stuck and also how it might feel to become free in specific areas of your life. This will give you a better idea of how much Aroma Freedom may benefit you, and where the best place will be for you to get started.

Personal Freedom and Fulfillment Check-in Exercise (For Everyone)

Before we proceed with the rest of the book, let's first check in with where you're at right now in terms of how emotionally free you feel right now.

Below, rate yourself on a scale from 1 - 5 on how accurate the statements are—1 means "not accurate at all," and 5 means "most accurate."

Once you've rated yourself for each statement, total up your scores and then use the Answer Key to determine your next steps.

Personal Freedom and Fulfillment Check-in Statement	Self-Rating
I work at a job (or am self-employed at a job) that I love	
I have a fulfilling relationship with a life partner, or am happy without one.	
I feel close and connected to people in my life	
I am at peace most days	
I love and accept myself, who I am, and what I have done	
I can think about events from the past freely,	

without being bothered by them	
I wake up each day with a sense of purpose and meaning	
I know that I am making a positive difference in the world	
I am able to express my wants and needs honestly and effectively	
I have activities in my life that I enjoy	
I feel healthy and energetic most of the time	
I am able to remain calm and peaceful even in the midst of stressful situations	
I know how I feel and what I want most of the time	
I feel a sense of personal empowerment in my life	
When strong feelings come over me, I feel confident that I can effectively deal with whatever is coming up	
I am able to feel and express anger appropriately, without feeling guilty afterwards	
I am able to feel sadness when I lose someone or something, without it ruining my whole day	
I am able to experience failure, or lose a game, without it ruining my whole day	

I rarely experience self-criticism, and when I do, I am able to learn how to improve myself	
I can hear criticism from others without becoming defensive or angry	
I know that my life has value and worth	
I can witness others' successes without becoming jealous	
I am able to pursue and achieve meaningful goals	
I am clear about what I want in life	
I am able to manifest the money I need for me and my family to live the way we would like to live	
I communicate with my partner and others in my life effectively	
TOTAL UP YOUR SCORE:	

What Your Score Really Means

> ### Score: 26 - 52
> ### Emotional Healing needs to become a Priority

If you have a low score on this exercise, it likely means that you are still carrying around quite a bit of baggage from unresolved emotional stressors and/or traumatic situations in your life. These unresolved situations make it difficult for you to function with the level of freedom that you desire. Your communication with others is likely inhibited, as is your ability to pursue and reach meaningful and fulfilling goals. This may also have a negative effect on your physical wellness and energy, and your financial situation.

However, the good news is that all of that can be fixed. Each of the above statements are reflective of the kinds of results people can experience with Aroma Freedom. By addressing these life areas individually through the Aroma Freedom process, you can begin to experience a "snowball" effect. As you become better able to navigate emotions in life, your work life will improve, your relationships will improve, and you will be on your way to a life of purpose and meaning.

As you read this book, pay attention to the stories of hope and healing from people just like you who have had powerful transformations and who have gone on to help others live happier, more meaningful lives. Try the exercises I give you in Part 3 so that you can experience this transformation firsthand, and follow the recommendations I give about how to begin or deepen your healing journey.

> ### Score: 53 - 78
> ### You are on the right track, keep growing!

If your score landed you here, it means that you likely have several areas in your life that are going pretty well. You may have a good job, close relationships, and some things in your life that bring you joy and happiness.

However, you probably also have some areas in your life that could benefit from additional improvement. Perhaps you have not yet found how to create the level of career or relationship fulfillment that you know you deserve. Or maybe you still find yourself thinking back to unhappy or unresolved memories and being overwhelmed with emotion. Or you worry about the future and are not sure how to face it.

With a good foundation of emotional health, you will probably be able to jump right in and fine-tune the areas of your life that are not working. Pay attention to the chapter on Aroma Freedom Technique and goal setting, and begin setting meaningful goals to work through using the processes in this book. Also, learn and practice the Aroma Reset (chapter 11) daily to raise your ability to handle the daily stresses of life.

> ### Score: 79+
> ### You are already flying...now let's soar!

If you have landed at this score, you likely have multiple areas in your life that are going really well. You are able to communicate effectively, set and reach goals, think about the past and future without becoming overwhelmed, and handle the stressors of life pretty well.

The next step for you would be to begin setting and reaching even bigger, more outrageous and fulfilling goals. Aiming your sights even higher will activate your true potential. It will also bring up any areas in your life that are still in need of healing, or where you are still limiting yourself.

As you read this book, pay attention to any inner voices coming up that believe that these results are "too good to be true." They may represent the final resistance your brain is putting up to stepping into the world of true accomplishment and joy. And, if you find yourself getting excited at the thought of helping yourself and others achieve this magical state of flow, you may want to explore becoming an Aroma Freedom Practitioner so that you can share this freedom with others.

Professional Fulfillment Check-in Exercise
(For Therapists, Coaches, and other Practitioners)

The previous exercise was for everyone, designed to assess personal freedom and fulfillment. If you have not yet done that exercise, please do it now before proceeding.

The exercise below is designed to help you assess how satisfied you are in your work as a coach or therapist. If you do not yet work in that field, you can skip this section.

Below, rate yourself on a scale from 1 - 5 on how accurate the statements are—1 means "not accurate at all," and 5 means "most accurate."

Once you've rated yourself for each statement, total up your scores and then use the Answer Key to determine your next steps.

Professional Fulfillment Check-in Statement	Self-Rating
I am excited to go into each session with a client	
I am confident that I will be able to help my client every time	
My clients almost always feel amazing at the end of the session	
I feel energized after working with clients	

I am comfortable with whatever comes up in a session with clients	
My clients report making positive changes in their lives regularly	
I am able to facilitate growth and transformation in a group format	
I am able to work just as effectively with my clients in-person or online	
Most of my sessions, even with complex clients, are pretty easy	
My clients are very grateful and appreciative of how I help them	
Clients frequently have life-changing sessions with me	
Clients often have major breakthroughs in how they view themselves, their history, and their life as a whole	
I know how to "clear" myself when I get triggered by something that comes up in a session	
I am able to help the client clear out memories without them having to tell me what the memory was about	
My clients become more confident, empowered, and goal-directed as they continue to work with me	

I have created workshops or courses that I lead people through in-person or online	
I have created evergreen courses that people can purchase with no additional work by me (i.e. passive income)	
I have developed a reputation as a leader in my field	
I love to learn new methods and integrate them into my own unique approach to coaching or therapy	
I am comfortable charging clients based on the transformation they receive	
I influence large numbers of people with the work I do, and continue to be excited to master my craft and reach even more people	
I am comfortable with marketing my services either in-person or online	
I am able to navigate new technologies as needed in order to establish my online presence	
I have integrated recent findings in neuroscience to enhance my offerings	
I like being the best practitioner I can be	
I have the support of family, friends and colleagues as I expand my business into new territory	

TOTAL UP YOUR SCORE:	

What Your Score Really Means

Score: 26 - 52
Professional Fulfillment has not yet occurred

If you have a low score on this exercise, it likely means that you are either new to your field, burned-out from doing the same thing for too long, or in need of additional training to allow you to become more effective and masterful in your practice. You may enjoy some aspects of your work, but are suffering in other parts. For instance, you may enjoy your practice but hate marketing it, or you love people but then get dragged into their pain and drama which in turn, drains you. You see that there is a lot of room for growth in your career.

This is not all bad, however. The fact that you see areas for possible growth could mean that this is the perfect time to learn something new and transformational. You will enjoy learning about the steps of Aroma Freedom and will become inspired by how quickly you may be able to learn this modality and bring it into your practice. If you choose to become certified, you can begin bringing this work to your clients in just a few months from now, and will be excited and amazed to see how quickly they progress.

If you also had a low score on the personal freedom and fulfillment exercise, it means that you will need to grow yourself in order to grow your business. This is exactly what happens when students turn into practitioners - they shed years of emotional baggage and have major emotional breakthroughs as they use and master the 6 Aroma Freedom Techniques. Then, as they bring this work into the world, they grow as a person while they are growing their business.

> Score: 53 - 78
> You love your work and are looking to improve your results

If your score landed you here, it means that you likely are getting good results with your clients, and yet you still see some areas for improvement. This could be in the realm of client results, or it could have to do with learning how to make your work less demanding of your energy. Perhaps you want to market yourself more effectively, or you want to bring your work to a larger audience.

In the pages that follow, pay attention to the aspects of Aroma Freedom that can impact your clients in ways that you have not yet been able to master. It could have to do with processing trauma more efficiently, teaching them how to manage stress better, or becoming better at goal-setting. If your struggles have to do with managing your own emotional energy, see how it feels to experience these techniques yourself and then translate that result for your clients.

For you, becoming certified in Aroma Freedom will be pretty straightforward. You have an existing client base that will love the techniques, and giving them even better results will raise your energy and make you more enthusiastic about expanding your offerings.

> **Score: 79+**
> **You are already successful - time to expand your influence**

If you have landed at this score, you likely have multiple areas in your practice that are going really well. You have mastered some techniques or approaches that work well for your clients, you enjoy what you do, and have achieved a level of financial success doing it. Congratulations!

Pay attention as you read this book to new ideas that come into your head about how you might be able to integrate Aroma Freedom into your existing offerings. This could be a module that you add to your coaching or treatment program, a new way to process trauma that is more gentle and efficient than what you are already using, or part of a class you want to create that can be sold as an additional stream of income.

When I teach Aroma Freedom to practitioners, I first require that they learn to deliver the process exactly as I teach it, without skipping steps or inserting their own tool into it. This way, they can learn exactly what Aroma Freedom can do all on its own. Once practitioners are certified, they are welcome to integrate the process into their own approach, or create an entirely new technique that is a synthesis of everything they do. I want my students to go beyond what I have done and create new things that reach more people - if you are an influencer and a life-changer, I invite you to learn these processes and watch how your mission gets even bigger with the addition of these tools.

What to expect:

When you begin using Aroma Freedom, you will be amazed at how quickly and gently it works. Memories that have troubled you for years or decades can be quickly processed and replaced by peace and equanimity. Current situations that you find overwhelming or frustrating will become manageable, even exciting to tackle. Goals and dreams that you desire personally or professionally will feel more within your reach. Worries about the unknown future will be replaced by wisdom for your life here and now.

If you are a coach or therapist, your work with clients will change radically. You will now have a tool you can use whenever your client is stuck or having a difficult time navigating their life. You will help them process traumatic or troubling memories quickly and gently, in a matter of minutes or hours, rather than months or years. You will feel energized by your work because of how efficient the process is. You will be able to help many people at once if you choose to do group sessions or classes, either in-person or online.

You will, however, need to be open to a new way of working that is radically simple and focused. In Aroma Freedom, we don't spend much time listening to clients' stories, or have them describe their trauma in detail. In each step of the Aroma Freedom process, as you will see in the coming chapters, we make a point to only get the information we need for the step at hand, before moving to the next step. This keeps the sessions moving quickly so we can get more done in one session than some therapies can accomplish in years! (Yes, I have had clients tell me this). In fact, here is a testimonial I found in my facebook group that was put up by one of my Certified Practitioners:

Teresa Hermann
May 26, 2018 · 🌐   •••

Just had to share this testimonial... "I have been in traditional psychotherapy for 2 decades (including Cognitive Behavioral Therapy) and had better results with Teresa in one session of AFT. Absolutely transformative! AFT is an amazing therapy, and I can't imagine a more compassionate or skillful guide to have on the journey than Teresa!" K.P. | Charlottesville, VA

👍❤️ You, Lisa Perkus Edmunds, Lynn Sullivan and 53 others   9 Comments

You will likely feel free to help more people, more quickly and deeply, and make more money (if you are a professional) than with your current set of tools. Even if you are not a helping professional, you will be inspired to share these tools with all of your friends, family, and colleagues, just so that they can have a taste of the freedom you will soon possess.

Key Chapter Takeaways

Personal freedom and fulfillment may include several areas, such as:

- Satisfying employment and relationships.
- Ability to tolerate and welcome all of the negative emotions that may surface in response to life events.
- Ability to feel joy and happiness.
- Freedom from guilt, shame, and self-criticism.
- Freedom to choose your own path.

Professional freedom and fulfillment as a therapist or coach may include:

- A sense of confidence and competence when working with clients.
- An understanding of how and why clients are stuck, and what to do about it.
- The ability to get consistently great results with clients.
- A method for processing trauma quickly and gently.
- The ability to work 1-1 or in groups.
- The ability to create courses that can help people all over the world, if desired.

Identifying where you have not yet found freedom can be a springboard to help you grow in new directions.

Chapter 4

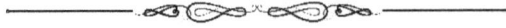

Why is Freedom and Fulfillment so Difficult to Attain?

(And How Aroma Freedom can Help)

Whether you are reading this book in order to solve your own problems or those of your clients, it is critical to first understand why personal growth and helping yourself or others is so difficult. I have been a Psychologist for over 20 years, and have seen many good hearted, intelligent people who suffered from depression, anxiety, PTSD, relationship problems, and more because they were not able to pull themselves out of the emotional rut they were in. Some of them had been on and off medications for years or had seen multiple therapists, and still had the same problems. Others had just suffered silently for decades, just "trying their best" to live a good life but still being plagued by these problems. Or, they had achieved a level of success in their lives, but it still felt empty and lacked a sense of meaning and purpose.

Why is freedom and fulfillment so difficult to attain? There are many ways to answer that question, but in this chapter, I will focus on three of the main causes of human unhappiness, why these are usually so hard to overcome, and how we handle them easily with Aroma Freedom. For each area, I will first discuss how it shows up in the quest for personal fulfillment, then I will show how this problem needs to be handled in your practice if you are a coach, therapist, or other helping professional.

1. Looking in the wrong place for the answer.

2. Getting lost in complexity.

3. Trying to build a new building on a crumbling foundation.

* * * * *

Obstacle #1 - Looking in the wrong place for the answer.

The well-known story that best sums up this phenomenon goes something like this:

You are taking a walk in the evening, and you see someone crawling on the ground under a street light, apparently looking for something. You ask if you can help.

"I've lost my keys," he says, "and I am looking for them."

"Where did you lose them?" you ask.

The man points across the street.

"I lost them over there," he says.

You think about this for a minute. "Well, if you lost them over there, why are you looking for them here?" you ask, with a confused look on your face.

"Because the light is better here," the man replies.

You scratch your head and walk away as he continues to look.

This story illustrates the problem of knowledge in general, and of self-knowledge and personal transformation in particular.

Most of the time, we can only see what our mindset, outlook, training, and experience has prepared us to see.

So, when you are trying to solve a problem on your own, you run into this limitation. You will approach every task, every problem, every challenge with the resources that you have developed over your lifespan. You will only look for solutions in the ways that make sense to you.

For instance, I worked with someone recently who had fallen into a pattern of social isolation (I will call her Sandy). She would putter around the house all day, starting and stopping cleaning projects, and eventually found herself not leaving the house, and not calling or interacting with people who she used to have good relationships with. She kept telling herself "today is the day I get up and leave the house." But then, nothing would happen.

I asked her why she thought she had this problem. She stated that she was probably just too busy and overwhelmed with her housework to make contact with her friends. She said that she must just be weak and that she should probably eat better so she would have more energy to do things like socialize. She would read books on willpower or nutrition to try to get up enough energy to interact with people, yet still she was not doing it.

I worked with her using the Aroma Freedom process, and the session went something like this:

Dr. Perkus: "Let's set a goal. What would you like to see happen in your life, but you are not sure if it will?" (This is how I start most AFT sessions)

Sandy: "My goal is to pick up the phone and call my niece. I love her but have been unable to pick up the phone for some reason."

Dr. Perkus: "How possible does that feel from 0-10."

Sandy: "I guess a 0 since I seem to never do it."

Dr. Perkus: "What does the negative voice in your head say, that tells you that you can't pick up the phone."

Sandy: "I hear a voice that sounds like my father's voice, telling me that nobody likes me and I should keep to myself." (She seems surprised to hear her father's voice - was not expecting that).

Dr. Perkus: "What emotion do you feel when you hear his voice saying that?"

Sandy: "Sad."

Dr. Perkus: "Where do you feel that sadness in your body?"

Sandy: "I feel it in my heart."

Dr. Perkus: "Connect with that feeling of sadness in your heart, and drift back to an earlier time when you felt the same way. Tell me when a memory pops up."

Sandy: "That's funny. I haven't thought of this in years…I am remembering a time when all of the neighborhood kids were playing outside, but my father told me not to go out there because they didn't like me." (She begins to tear up).

I put a drop of "Inner Child" essential oil blend into her hand and asked her to breathe the aroma into the memory and notice what happened.

As she did this, it unlocked a flood of other memories related to her father, including scenes of physical abuse, drunken rage, and her feeling scared and angry.

We used the Aroma Freedom process to clear out these memories, thoughts and feelings, each time having her smell specific oils, and notice what happened.

(I will give you the details about the steps of the exact techniques, as well as which essential oils we use in the next section).

After about 15 minutes, she put her hands down and looked at me, amazed.

Sandy: "I just forgave my father for the first time," she said with a combination of awe, confusion, and gratitude.

She explained that her alcoholic father had been very cruel and abusive when she was young, and she had tried, through years of therapy and self-help, to come to peace with him but would always feel a combination of sadness, hurt, and terror when she thought of him. This had been going on for 60+ years (she was 75 when I began working with her, and her abuse had occurred as a young child).

Yet somehow, through this brief Aroma Freedom process, not only did the negative feelings about her father go away, but she felt compassion for him and was able to see the world through his eyes. She was shocked that these memories had surfaced, because her father had been dead for over a decade, and her current predicament seemingly had nothing to do with him.

Dr. Perkus: "How possible does it feel now to call your niece?"

Sandy: (Her face lighting up and a smile coming onto her face). "I know I can call her now. I am realizing now that I have always approached conversations with the sense that maybe they don't really want to talk to me. Now I can imagine calling her and I don't hear that voice. Instead, I have the feeling that she will be happy to talk to me!"

This story illustrates several important points.

1. This client assumed that her disinclination to leave the house had something to do with either lack of energy, low willpower, or overwhelm, because those were the

only explanations that came to her mind (She was looking in the wrong place for the answer).

2. The real cause of the problem was locked away in her subconscious brain in memories that were 60+ years old. They were not visible because they were shrouded in the darkness of time, and her conscious mind would never have assumed that these memories could connect with her current problem.

The Aroma Freedom process is revolutionary because it enables us to consistently find the root causes to many of the most vexing problems we encounter. As you will see in part 2 of this book, Aroma Freedom works in such a way that hidden memories and connections spontaneously emerge that hold the keys to why we think, feel, or act a certain way. Even more importantly, however, we are then enabled to quickly and gently dismantle these now revealed "memory complexes" so that we can once again pursue our lives in the direction of our dreams.

In your own life, think of any annoying or self-destructive habits you have, any dreams you want to pursue but somehow don't, any relationship or personal problems you have been unable to solve. Do you know where to look to find the answers? Do you have confidence that you can figure it out on your own? How has that worked so far?

For now, take a moment to check in with yourself.

"Looking in the wrong place"
Personal Check-in Exercise

Before we proceed with the rest of the book, let's first check in with where you're at right now with knowing how to solve personal problems.

Below, rate yourself on a scale from 1 - 5 on how accurate the statements are—1 means "not accurate at all," and 5 means "most accurate."

Once you've rated yourself for each statement, total up your scores and then use the Answer Key to determine your next steps.

Personal Problems Check-in Statement	Self-Ra ting
When I am stuck or confused, I know exactly what to do to find answers.	
I am able to easily break self-destructive habits and behaviors.	
I have stopped reading book after book on self-help because I have a reliable method for solving my problems.	
When I feel like a project is stalled out, I am able to get going in the right direction again quickly.	

The deeper roots of my problems become clear to me quickly when I go to solve them.	
When I find myself in a dark or negative mood, I am able to quickly decode the wisdom hidden within the mood and shift into a more positive place.	
I find setting and reaching goals to be fun and rewarding.	
I am able to easily break overwhelming tasks into simple processes and then take inspired action.	
When I find myself thinking about upsetting memories, I immediately begin clearing the memory in order to create resolution and find guidance in my current life situation.	
I get excited when I discover a part of my life that is not working the way I want, because it becomes a fun and interesting project of self-discovery.	
I have ceased blaming others for my problems, and turn instead to find the hidden roots for unpleasant situations within my own consciousness.	
TOTAL UP YOUR SCORE:	

What Your Score Really Means

Score: 11 - 20
You are flailing without a lifejacket

If your score falls into this range, it is likely that you really don't have a lot of tools to pull you through the challenges of solving your personal problems. You probably have some self-destructive habits, feel overwhelmed much of the time, and generally feel lost when you are facing many of the problems in life.

If this is you, you are not alone. Life on earth can be very complex, and many of us are just not equipped with the tools to move in the direction we want to go. When we feel this way, we become desperate for solutions. Sometimes this can land us in a dysfunctional relationship, whether with a romantic partner, boss, or even a well-meaning but misguided friend who promises to solve our problems for us.

You may struggle with food or other addictions, be not as productive as you think you should be, and in general feel that you are not reaching your true potential. Don't worry! In the following pages I will be describing some very simple yet powerful techniques you can use right away to begin decoding and dealing with even your most daunting personal challenges. These processes are able to be used by yourself, or if you feel too overwhelmed to use them alone then I will show you how to find additional help in applying them to your own life.

Score: 21 - 35
Getting a grip most of the time

If you fall into this group, congratulations! You likely have a pretty good ability to solve your own problems by getting to the root of the issue even when it is not obvious. You might be doing this by following a system or technique that works for you, talking to a wise coach, therapist, or friend, or have just gained wisdom over the years of trial and error.

The challenge at this level is to be able to consistently push yourself beyond your comfort zone and embrace more and more challenging projects. It is human nature to settle into a certain degree of mastery and not realize how much further you could actually grow yourself.

With Aroma Freedom, the goal setting process is designed to keep us reaching and stretching beyond what we know we can do, so that we can see how far we can go. And you will be surprised, when you try it, at just how quickly you will go from feeling that a goal or dream is out of reach, to feeling confident and excited about achieving it. Pay attention in section 2 when I discuss the goal setting process and why we formulate goals the way that we do.

Score: 35+
Mastery...but can you help others?

You are masterful in solving problems in most areas of your life. Now the question is to determine how well you are able to help others solve their problems too. Helping others is a natural extension of feeling pretty satisfied with one's own abilities. After all, it is no fun to feel happy and content with your life when those around you are miserable!

I created Aroma Freedom with exactly this goal in mind - to create a process that is easy to do and to teach, so that success and happiness could be transferred from one person to another. Now that you have learned how to solve your own problems and find answers when you need them, would you like to learn some simple ways to help others as well? Then keep reading and pay attention when I discuss the neuroscience behind how this all works - this will show you that the basis for this process does not lie in luck or simply being blessed with a powerful personality, but it is truly something within reach for anyone who desires to use it.

How does Obstacle #1 show up for Coaches and Therapists?

Remember when I said above that Obstacle #1 was: **Looking in the wrong place for the answer.**

This rule obviously applies to Coaches and Therapists as much as to individuals.

For Coaches and Therapists, or any helping professional, the limit to their ability to help is defined by their "model of help" that they have been trained to use. Every helping professional has training and experience that guides how they approach each client.

For instance, if you are a Cognitive-Behavioral Therapist, you have been trained to look for and identify the negative subconscious thoughts that create all kinds of problems for your client. And you have been taught many methods for countering those thoughts, such as challenging the irrationality of the thoughts, distracting from the thoughts, substituting positive thoughts in their place, etc. The success you have with your clients is proportional to how well these methods work, and how compliant your clients are in doing their homework, etc.

Or, perhaps you are a coach that works with clients to help them get a broad overview of the areas in their life that are working, and the areas that are not working. Then you help them set goals for creating greater success in those areas that they want to improve, and you act as an accountability partner to make sure that they stay on track until they complete their goals. Again, the success you have will be related to how well your clients can stay on track in the goal achievement process.

Obstacle #1 comes into play for these professionals when the methods they are using just aren't working for some of their clients. In these cases it is common and even understandable to blame the client. After all, if they just did their homework, or followed through on their action steps, they would be doing great! So why aren't they?

If you, as a helping professional, don't know how to uncover the **hidden determinants** of behavior, you will feel stuck and frustrated with these clients. You will feel that no matter how you approach their problems, there is something else that is stopping your clients from succeeding. And, you will be correct in that assumption!

Through facilitating and observing thousands of hours of work with Aroma Freedom, I am continually amazed at how the hidden traumas, memories, and subconscious thought processes rise to the surface in surprising and unexpected ways, and suddenly what was a mystery becomes crystal clear. When a person will not or can not change despite their own sincere desire to do so, it means that there is some hidden root that has yet to be uncovered. Once it rises to the surface and is cleared, the desired change seems to almost magically happen.

In Graduate school at Duquesne University, I was trained in the philosophical and psychological approach of "Phenomenology." One of the core tenets of this view is to "make no assumptions" about a thing, but rather, to let it show itself from itself, through careful observation. This could only be accomplished through a disciplined approach on the part of the observer, taking care to question one's assumptions and not to insert a theory about a thing that might get in the way of observing what it actually is.

When I created Aroma Freedom, I used the same approach, and as you will see in part 2, it is critical to follow the steps of the approach and not to insert your own theories about what you will find. Rather, you need to leave your assumptions about the hidden cause of the behavior "at the door," and let the true roots of the problem show themselves and be cleared.

"Looking in the Wrong Place"
Professional Check-in Exercise

The first check-in in this chapter was for everyone. The one below is mainly for Professional Coaches, Therapists, or other Helping Professionals. If this does not describe you, feel free to skip this survey.

For this survey, let's check in with where you're at now in your ability to get to the root of your client's problems.

Below, rate yourself on a scale from 1 - 5 on how accurate the statements are—1 means "not accurate at all," and 5 means "most accurate."

Once you've rated yourself for each statement, total up your scores and then use the Answer Key to determine your next steps.

Professional Problem Solving Check-in Statement	Self-Ratin g
I know how to quickly get to the root of my clients' underlying problems.	
I get excited when my client tells me that they are stumped as to why they can't get results, because I know I will find something new with my methods.	
When clients are not compliant with what I have	

asked them to do, I get really curious instead of frustrated.	
I am totally comfortable with starting a session having no idea where it will go, because I know the system will guide me.	
When strong emotions come up in a session, I am able to easily guide the client on how to break through to a state of peace and freedom.	
I am able to put all of my theories aside when working with a client, in order to discover what is really happening with them.	
I am willing to not be the "expert" in the session, but rather to help the client break through to the inner awareness of their own wisdom and guidance.	
I am willing to let go of the "surface story" the client is telling, in order for their deeper truth to emerge.	
I am able to maintain my calm and equanimity in each session, because I am not being flooded with their traumatic stories.	
I find my work to be fun, rewarding, and energizing.	
I am regularly surprised and delighted by the wisdom my clients spontaneously receive from their intuition during our sessions.	
I am inspired to keep growing as a practitioner	

when I see my clients have amazing breakthroughs regularly.	
My clients thank me profusely for helping them reach their highest potential.	
I am planning or am currently providing group sessions or classes to reach more people with my work.	
TOTAL UP YOUR SCORE:	

What Your Score Really Means

> **Score: 14 - 24**
> **Just getting started**

With a score in the lower ranges, it means that you have not yet found a way to consistently move from the surface presentation of clients problems, to the depths where the root causes lie. You get caught chasing their symptoms around, looking for solutions but not really finding them. You are frequently stumped when your clients don't improve as fast as they or you would like them to.

You are in need of a reliable roadmap to the human emotional landscape, a guide that will show you how to find hidden causes that are not obvious. You are looking for solutions based on what you have been taught in graduate school or coach training, but this has not yet translated into reliable results for your clients.

To course-correct and improve your practice, keep reading these pages. In the next few chapters, you will find a remarkably simple and yet profound approach that works with all kinds of problems, helping you to consistently deliver breakthrough sessions for your clients that will leave them amazed and grateful, and will leave you energized and inspired. Don't give up!

Score: 25 - 36
You are getting good…keep learning!

You have been practicing your craft long enough to become proficient at helping clients achieve breakthroughs and significant changes. You aren't fooled by the surface presentation that clients bring, and are able to apply skills and techniques that are making a real difference in clients lives. You enjoy what you do and love to keep learning how to become better at it.

You may still be missing out on some opportunities to help clients make even more significant, quick, or lasting changes, however. Perhaps you still get caught up in their stories, or keep pushing them down a path that is not quite the right one for them. They may still be leaning on you as the expert rather than learning how to listen to their own intuition for guidance.

As you read about the Aroma Freedom Techniques in the following pages, think about your current clients and how these approaches might be able to help them. Because you love to learn, you will probably enjoy the opportunity to bring something new to them and see how much better your results might be.

Score: 37+
Time To Duplicate Yourself

You are already doing amazing work with your clients.

Congratulations! This has probably come through many years of training, practice, and experience. You may have a natural gift for sniffing out hidden causes and the inner working of things. Yet there could still be an area that you have not yet developed, and that is the ability to teach your clients how to do what you do.

That may sound a little strange. How or why would a coach or therapist want to teach their client how to be like them? Doesn't that defeat the purpose of being a practitioner?

Remember the saying, "Give a man a fish and you feed him for a day. Teach him to fish, and you feed him for life?"

Ultimately, we don't want our clients to keep coming to us forever. We want them to go off and lead productive, independent lives.

But in order to teach them how to solve their own problems, we need a system.

That is where Aroma Freedom really shines.

Because it is a system that is easily taught and duplicated, it is ideal as a tool that can be handed from practitioner to client, from teacher to student, on and on.

The reason that I left my successful Psychology practice in 2016 is because I realized that I was helping more people by teaching the The Aroma Freedom Technique online to people all across the world, than I could ever help by meeting with them 1-1 in my office, day after day.

If you are already masterful as a coach or therapist, I would love to show you how using Aroma Freedom can give you a duplicatable skill that you can teach your most devoted clients to help them become even more independent and successful. In the certification program we discuss how to create classes and group experiences for clients that teach them these skills so that they can continue to grow beyond us. You will be able to leverage your time by serving more people in this way, making more money and impact in the process.

If this describes you and you are already feeling the pull to create this lasting impact, go ahead and book a call with us at www.aromafreedom.com/call and we will discuss your situation to see if training is right for you.

Obstacle #2 - Getting lost in complexity.

Many of our problems seem too complex to understand and solve. Just as in the last section, Sandy had her theories about why she was not initiating contact with loved ones...but they were all wrong! We often spin our wheels trying to find solutions, when the answer may be under our nose all the time! (Pun intended - this is a book about Aroma after all :)

In the following section, I will describe why humans are so complex, and discuss an example of a problem that has been made complex by the way our brains work. We will look at how traditional approaches deal with this complexity through equally complex solutions. Then, I will show you how Aroma Freedom can deal with the same problem, but very **simply**. Once you see how simple it can be to deal with many of the problems you walk around with, your sense of freedom will grow and you will be able to get to the heart of your problems (or those of your clients) much more quickly. You will also see how aromatherapy fits into all of this - how our most primal sense of **smell** can be used to cut through the complexity created by our less sensory-bound cerebral cortex.

So, where does all of this complexity come from?

Human beings are amazing creatures. Evolution (or Intelligent Design, depending on your beliefs) has gifted us with a large neocortex in our brain, which enables us to do incredibly complex things, such as language, music, imagination, engineering, mathematics, planning, and so much more. In fact, most of what we see when we look at modern civilization is only possible because of our large cerebral cortex. When compared with other animals, the difference in size and complexity of the brain is huge, and this corresponds to the difference between human society and, let's say, chimpanzee society. Chimps can use some basic tools, can learn a few dozen symbols when communicating with researchers, but otherwise they don't go around building computers, skyscrapers, or writing symphonies like humans do.

Humans have the ability to imagine a future that has not yet arrived. We will create theories, narratives, and conjectures about practically everything that has not yet happened. We will also ruminate endlessly about what has <u>already</u> happened. So here we sit, lost in the past or the future, while the present moment is the only time in which anything can actually take place. The time for action is always now, yet so often we don't act because of all of the considerations about past and future.

Everything we experience becomes a memory. The more novel, intense, or emotionally charged it was, the more likely we are to remember it. We remember events not as they occurred, but according to what they meant to us, then and now. This is why we will rehash the past, going over all of the things that did or did not happen, and what they meant.

When we consider our future, we do the same thing. Except instead of picturing and thinking about past events, we create, through our extraordinary powers of imagination, a future that may or may not ever come to pass.

This is why our lives are so complicated. We have thousands of past experiences to mull over and consider as we choose from thousands of possible futures.

Now take an everyday example. Let's say a young man wants to ask a girl on a date. When he is thinking of approaching her, there are a million things running through his mind. He is imagining her reaction - Will she say yes? Will she laugh at him? Will she make up a lame excuse? Will others laugh at him? As he considers this, he is taking into account his previous experiences - what has happened in the past when he has approached girls? What has he seen happen to his friends? What has he seen in movies and on TV? All of these experiences filter into what he imagines will happen when he approaches her. Past and Imagined Future are all in play as he approaches.

"Hi, would you like to go out with me sometime?"

"Um, I would love to but sorry my mother does not let me date."

He walks away and his head is spinning even more now.

His thoughts go something like this:

"Is that the truth or did she just make it up to get away from me?"

"Who can I ask to see if that is true?"

"Do I know any of her friends?"

"But would they tell her if I asked them?"

"Maybe they are all laughing at me right now behind my back."

Now he is imagining them all laughing at him.

He never approaches her again.

Years go by, and he thinks back to that time when he really liked a girl, asked her out, and she said no.

He remembers all of her friends were laughing at him as he walked away.

The fact that he never actually saw her laughing with her friends gets forgotten. Now what he imagined is part of the memory.

How does this man, now an adult, approach relationships? He has memories from high school that do not support him being confident now. His lack of confidence leads to social withdrawal, isolation, and eventually depression.

When faced with a problem like this to solve, where should he even start? There are probably a hundred other things to take into account, such as what life was like in his family, other experiences he had with his friends and siblings, his basic personality structure, conversations he has had with friends, teachers, parents, and so much more.

Eventually he comes into therapy or he seeks out some life coaching, to try to get back on track. Unfortunately, there is a chance that the therapist or coach may get just as confused as he is as to how to solve his problem. Normally, the practitioner will do one of two things, or a combination:

1. **Supportive counseling.** In this case, simply having a compassionate, empathic person to talk to could be helpful for him. Over time, he may get more comfortable expressing himself in therapy and eventually in real life. He may slowly build up his confidence, try again, and perhaps even succeed in developing a relationship.

2. **Structured Therapy or Coaching.** There are many forms of therapy and coaching, each based on a theory of what motivates human beings to do what they do. Many of them are effective. They may find and challenge his negative thoughts, they may help him process negative memories, they may hold him accountable to make small steps each week, etc. One thing they all have in common, however, is that they work to untangle the web of beliefs, thoughts, feelings, and experiences that make him who he is.

Becoming a therapist or coach usually requires years of training, experience, and supervision, because as I have been mentioning in this chapter, humans are extraordinarily complex. Untangling the web of their suffering is hard work.

Most efforts to solve emotional problems, whether by oneself or with the help of a therapist or coach, are hindered by the complexity we have been discussing.

On one hand, we have therapies that attempt to understand where the problem is coming from. They do this by taking a detailed history, getting information about one's family, childhood experiences, and so on, and then creating a map of how the person got into such a mess and how to get out of it. The advantage of this approach is that by understanding the past we are in a better position, theoretically at least, to learn from it and do something different now. The disadvantage of this approach is that it is possible to become stuck in the past, and never actually get to create the dreamed-of future. This is the scenario where people are in therapy for years.

On the other hand, we have some therapies, and most coaching approaches, that dispense with looking into the past altogether and just focus on the future - on setting and achieving goals. This could be called solution-focused therapy, brief therapy, accountability coaching, or something similar. The advantage of this approach is that, by focusing on the future, we don't get bogged down in the complexities of the past. The disadvantage is that sometimes we can't move forward because we are carrying too much weight in the form of unresolved trauma and dysfunctional beliefs rooted in trauma. These subconscious beliefs actually hinder and even sabotage progress until they are dealt with (like my belief that I was not strong enough to finish, as mentioned in chapter 1).

The best therapies and coaching approaches, then, would be ones that integrate both a past and a future focus, without getting lost in either. Navigating between past and future is what gets complicated and why becoming masterful in therapy or coaching takes so long. It is also why, until now, it has been nearly impossible to do on one's own.

The Aroma Freedom Solution to Complexity

In Part 2 of this book, I will show you exactly what Aroma Freedom is in greater detail, how it is used, and why it can accomplish so much in so little time. The short version is this: Aroma Freedom takes the basic structure of everything mentioned above - i.e. focusing on the future while clearing out the past - and does it all in **each session**.

Every Aroma Freedom session has a beginning, a middle, and an end.

In the **beginning** phase of the session, you focus your attention on a goal and how possible it feels that you can attain it. The goal setting part of the session is critical because it will set the tone for everything else that happens. When you set a goal, something very interesting happens in your brain. You immediately go about assessing how likely it will be that you can reach the goal. Any negative thoughts you have been harboring will come to the surface. The goal setting can take as little as 1 minute (if you are already very clear on what you want) to as much as 15 minutes or more (if you really don't know what you want).

In the **middle** phase of the session, you take some time to identify the negative thoughts, feelings, and memories that have gotten triggered by setting the goal. Then you clear them out using the power of aroma with specific essential oil blends (see the Appendix at the end of this book for guidance on which oils we use). You do as many rounds of this as you need until, when you think of the goal, there is nothing within you that says it cannot happen. Instead, you feel energized, excited and hopeful about your prospects. This usually takes 10-40 minutes, depending on how many negative thoughts and memories there are.

In the **end** phase of the session, you consolidate the newfound positive attitude or mindset you have created and form either an affirmation or a question that will help you to remain focused on the actions needed to complete your goal. You anchor this mindset with the essential oils.

This 3-part structure is baked in to every session, and it reduces complexity in several ways:

1. In the beginning phase of the session, rather than taking a long, detailed history of the problem, we jump right into goal setting. This allows you to bypass the endless complexity of the pre-history of the problem. So much of the time, we get lost telling our story, explaining why we think we have these problems. The reality of the situation is that we don't really know why we have our problems. If we did, we probably wouldn't have the problem. To reiterate what was mentioned earlier, we usually are looking in the wrong place for the solution.

2. In the middle phase of the session, we allow our own subconscious chatter to lead us right back to the memories that are most connected to the obstacle we are seeking to overcome. Rather than creating theories

about which traumas or unpleasant experiences or thoughts are interfering with problem resolution, we let that emerge organically through the Aroma Freedom process. It is very quick and to-the-point. Once we have identified the triggering memories, we breathe essential oils into the memory complex and, due to the immediacy of the sense of smell, the memories change and resolve very quickly (in a matter of seconds or minutes, not weeks or months as in traditional counseling). This speed of memory processing is one of the prime areas that sets Aroma Freedom apart from almost every other method for dealing with the past. The full process of Memory Reconsolidation that occurs, as well as which essential oils we use, will be explained in part 2 of this book.

3. In the end phase of the session, we take advantage of the new positive mindset to move right into affirming action steps that will most quickly get us on the path of achieving our goal. Because there is no longer a negative voice telling us that what we want is impossible, this allows action to be inspired, efficient, and effective.

People have told us many times that 1 session has helped them more than years of therapy. This makes sense: You can spend years looking for your keys under the streetlight and never be successful, or you can spend minutes looking for them where you lost them and find them right away! The Aroma Freedom shows you where to look - and when you find the key, you can quickly unlock the door you were meaning to go through.

Struggling with Complexity Check-in Exercise

Let's do a quick check in with where you're at right now in your struggle with complexity.

Below, rate yourself on a scale from 1 - 5 on how accurate the statements are—1 means "not accurate at all," and 5 means "most accurate."

Once you've rated yourself for each statement, total up your scores and then use the Answer Key to determine your next steps.

"Struggling with Complexity" Check-in Statement	Self Rating
I have lots of theories about my problems but few solutions.	
Everyone I talk to about my problems gives me different answers and recommendations.	
I have read many books about psychology or self-help yet still struggle to find deep solutions.	
I am overwhelmed when trying to sort through all of the information about what to do.	
I have seen therapists or coaches for years but don't make much progress.	
I am tired of talking about my problems and not	

getting anywhere.	
TOTAL UP YOUR SCORE:	

What Your Score Really Means

Score: 22 - 30
You are fed up by complexity

If your score falls into this range, it is likely that you have been trying for years to get answers to some basic problems in your life and have been frustrated. You may have a tendency to overthink, and this creates problems because each thought generates 10 more thoughts, and pretty soon you feel like you're spinning your wheels and not getting anywhere.

Pay attention to the section on "Naming Feelings" in part 2 - this will show you a quick way to cut through the chatter and identify what is really going on underneath all of the complexity you are experiencing.

Score: 12 - 21
Some complexity, some peace

If you fall into this group, it means that you still experience some level of frustration with complexity, but you also have peace in some areas. It may or may not be an everyday problem, but there is likely at least one area in your life that you have been stumped in your efforts to move forward. You do possess some ability to cut through the noise and keep things simple. The goal for you now would be to keep working to reduce complexity, or to solve a major problem that has been thwarting

101

you.

> **Score: Less than 11**
> **Zen master**

You have been able to solve major life problems and possess an excellent ability to get to the heart of issues without chasing multiple concepts and theories around. Congratulations! You will really enjoy the simplicity of Aroma Freedom and how quickly it works to simplify. It will be a tool you can use with family and friends to help them to become as peaceful as you are!

Jenny Mehler
August 29 at 11:11 PM · 😊

I continue to be humbled and honored to lead Aroma Freedom sessions and be a witness to the incredible emotional and spiritual healing that can occur with this technique!

I led a session last week that was simply beautiful and provided a new layer of release, forgiveness, and healing for a client who experienced trauma as a child. I've had a few sessions with her over the last year or two, and the progress she's made has been awesome.

However, she recently experienced a major setback when a friend of hers asked if she could practice a different, very popular modality with her (similar to how we practitioners practice AFT before we are certified). It left her feeling very raw and vulnerable, almost like she'd experienced a "spiritual attack", she said, and she needed help processing it.

It was an incredibly moving healing session - definitely Holy Spirit led, I'm convinced! Her affirmation was divinely inspired. She felt like she was finally free! In the session, she had not only been forgiven by her inner child, she felt completely whole, and unconditionally loved!

As I continue to lead sessions like these, I feel I am finally stepping into my higher purpose. From the bottom of my heart (and from my client as well!), Thank you, so much, Dr. Benjamin Perkus, for creating and sharing this technique with us!

💜 🙏

Obstacle #3 - Trying to build a new building on a crumbling foundation.

When we want to make changes in our lives, we tend to gravitate towards solutions that "add" something. If you are lonely, add a relationship. If you are broke, add a job. If you are overweight, add a workout routine. This works some of the time, but it can also cause as many problems as it solves.

Obviously, trying to "add" a relationship when you are already in one is a recipe for disaster. Adding a new job when you already have one could lead to overwork and burnout. Adding a workout routine could be a good idea, but if you have unhealthy eating habits or other unresolved health issues, you could be setting yourself up for injury or worse.

In short, before you add something, make sure there isn't something that isn't working that needs to be removed or altered first. This bit of common sense may seem obvious, but when we get into the science of personal transformation in part 2 of this book, you will see that when we ignore this dictum (subtract before you add), our results will suffer.

Let's take a more concrete example. Remember our lonely friend from earlier in this chapter who had a bad experience when asking out a girl in high school? Imagine that he is now in his 20's and is in therapy because he feels isolated and lonely. The therapist talks with him about doing things to get him more "out there" like joining a social club or a softball team. This seems like a fair suggestion, except for one problem:

The young man will be carrying the same lack of confidence from his perceived rejection years ago, into the current situation. He will mumble when talking to these new potential friends, he will stand to the side and not participate in their banter, he will interpret even the slightest lack of attention from them as a deliberate snub.

In this case, the therapist is trying to help the young man to build a new building (fun social life) on top of a crumbling foundation (unresolved memory of rejection from high school). [1]

By not understanding this point, the young man will have to struggle against his tendency to want to withdraw. The therapist or coach will have to apply pressure to get him to follow through, because each time he thinks of going to the social club he gets a knot in his stomach. This is the very definition of mental and emotional conflict - One part of him wants to engage with others and be social, another part wants to go hide under a rock.

In fact, this is the primary struggle involved in all attempts to change: Inner Division

When we are divided (one part of us wants to change and another part doesn't), this leads to two problems:

---

[1] NOTE: This example is of course simplistic. There are usually multiple memories or negative incidences that would go into forming a globalized belief system. But the principle will still remain, that early life experiences will create beliefs that influence later life, unless and until they are changed and re-written.

1. Change is very difficult because we are fighting with ourselves.

2. Change is unstable and not long-lasting, because, even after making a change, there is a chance we could revert back to our former state.

This is easy to imagine in the case of addiction, for instance. When people try to give up smoking, drinking, or overeating, the most common pattern is flip-flopping between giving up the substance for a period of time, only to take it up once again (often with a vengeance). It usually requires a deeper transformation of the person (by hitting "rock bottom," or by a deep re-alignment of values) for such changes to actually be permanent ones. Even then, there may still be a struggle to maintain the new state.

Luckily, the brain has ways of rewriting the meaning of past events so that they no longer have the same hold on us. We could easily imagine that our lonely young man did eventually go to the social club, and he felt accepted by them and enjoyed himself, gradually coming out of his shell. In this case, he was able to develop new beliefs about being welcomed, loved, accepted, etc. In the best case scenario, this led him to being able to have a satisfying social life going forward. We could also imagine partial success - he is able to make some friends and relationships, but still has the nagging feeling that he is not really welcome or accepted.

Memory Reconsolidation refers to the natural brain process by which we are able to re-write the meaning of emotionally charged memories such that they are no longer bothersome. We will discuss this process in a later chapter. For now, it is important to realize that Memory Reconsolidation is involved whenever a person "gets over" a traumatic event - whenever they are able to deeply change how the past event has affected them. Importantly, Aroma Freedom fulfills all of the requirements of Memory Reconsolidation and is one of the best and fastest means to achieve this change.

Here is how an Aroma Freedom session might go with our lonely, isolated young man (abbreviated version):

AFT: "What would you like to accomplish in the session today?"

Man: "My goal is to have a fulfilling social life."

AFT: "OK, when you say and picture that, how possible does it feel (from 0-10, where 0=hopeless and 10=totally confident)"

Man: "Maybe a 5"

AFT: "OK, say your goal and listen in - what does the negative voice say that tells you this cannot happen?"

Man: "It says - 'They'll laugh at you.'"

AFT: "How do you feel when you hear that voice?"

Man: "Embarrassed."

AFT: "Where do you feel that embarrassment in your body?"

Man: "My eyes look downward and my cheeks feel flushed."

AFT: "OK. Close your eyes and drift back to an earlier time when you felt the same way."

Man: "I see myself in high school. I had just asked Becky Dodd out and she said no, then I turned around and knew that her friends were all laughing at me."

AFT: "OK, here are some essential oils. Put a drop on your hand and cup your hands and breathe the scent into that memory. Keep doing that for a minute or two, until you notice something has changed." (Stay tuned for Part 2 where I explain how this all works).

Man: (after a minute) "I see the image fading...they seem far away, all her friends have gone away...I turn around and see her smiling at me. I can tell that she liked me too but she just couldn't go with me."

AFT: "Yes. Now say your goal again, and rate how possible it feels now."

Man: "It feels like a 9 or 10. I feel excited to go and make friends. Somehow I just don't feel as tongue tied or embarrassed any more."

(Session continues with follow-up actions, etc. See Section 2 for detailed instructions of a full session.)[2]

---

[2] This simplified excerpt of a sample Aroma Freedom session is not far from what actually happens in each session. If this were a real session, we would have spent some more time formulating the goal. And, there may have been a few more rounds of memories to clear, but each would have followed the same pattern - name the goal, trace the negative voice back to

What just happened in this session was **Memory Reconsolidation.** A memory was accessed in its full emotional, cognitive, and bodily expression, and then, by breathing specific essential oils into the image, the memory itself transformed. This is not just a fantasy or wishful thinking - those who have experienced this will tell you that the memory itself is different after such a process. Many times they cannot even remember what the memory was like before it had shifted.

Once the memory reconsolidated, there was a spontaneous positive image and message that emerged from the memory. This is one of the most amazing things about the Aroma Freedom process. After the memory transforms, there is usually a positive message that the person becomes aware of. This is not something that can be predicted - it is unique to the individual and seems to represent a form of "inner guidance" or "inner wisdom" that arises on its own.

When the memory is processing, most people notice the memory visually change - it breaks apart, gets further away, or fades out. Sometimes it fades completely to the point where it is not visible at all. Sometimes it does not change visually but the emotional charge is gone - they can look at the memory and not feel strong emotion any more.

For some people, it involves a change in what actually happens in the memory. I remember one student I worked with as a demonstration (in front of 300 people, no less!) who had the

---

the memory, breathe essential oils into the image until it dissolves, return to the goal until there are no more negative voices.

following experience: She had related that her mother had been very abusive to her as a child, and at times would tell her to clean her room. And if the child did not clean it fast enough, the mother would throw all of the clothes and toys on the floor and make her clean it again.

After having activated this traumatic memory, I had her breathe essential oils into the memory. A few minutes later, she smiled, and said that as she continued to breathe the oils into the memory, the memory changed and became like a scene out of "Mary Poppins." She could see the clothes and toys being magically flown back into their proper place in the closet and drawers. As this happened her tears stopped, her mood lifted, and she received a message something like: "This was the only thing my mother knew how to do - it wasn't about me. I am free now."

The important thing in all of these examples is not so much about what happens visually to the memory, but what the new, positive message is. Once the message is received, the memory takes on a completely new meaning, and the person becomes free to pursue his or her goals without hearing a nagging inner voice telling them that it is not possible.

How does all of this relate to the problem under discussion, namely, **Trying to build a new building on a crumbling foundation?**

Well, the foundation is the life we have lived up to this point, including the memories, beliefs, expectations, attitudes, habits, etc. These form the basis from which we will approach any new venture - such as forming a relationship, building a business, maintaining our health, parenting our kids, and so on. We will do what our past experience + our beliefs tell us is the thing to be done. If our foundation is full of holes, such as poor self-esteem, bad habits, negative expectations, then the building we are attempting to create will have these same holes in it.

The discovery of Memory Reconsolidation and the fact that Aroma Freedom can facilitate it so quickly and easily has created a whole new possibility in the realm of personal transformation, whether it be administered in the form of self-help, therapy, or coaching.

By going back and "clearing up" the past, this creates the opportunity to create a new life for the person going forward, based on the person's goals, dreams, and values, rather than continuing to live within the self-imposed limitations that were created when they were a child first navigating the world. Aroma Freedom can help us to build our future on a solid foundation.

Building on a Solid Foundation Check-in Exercise

Let's do a quick check in with where you're at right now in your efforts to resolve the past and build your life on a solid foundation going forward.

Below, rate yourself on a scale from 1 - 5 on how accurate the statements are—1 means "not accurate at all," and 5 means "most accurate."

Once you've rated yourself for each statement, total up your scores and then use the Answer Key to determine your next steps.

"Building on a Solid Foundation" Check-in Statement	Self Rating
I feel complete with the past.	
I believe in myself and know I can accomplish what I set out to do.	
I have life-supportive habits that give me plenty of energy to pursue my goals and dreams.	
I am able to accept criticism and ask for help when needed.	
I am able to feel an appropriate level of pride in my accomplishments.	
I am able to give and receive love.	

I am connected to my intuition or to a higher power for guidance.	
TOTAL UP YOUR SCORE:	

What Your Score Really Means

Score: 7 - 16
Your foundation is shaky

If your score falls into this range, it is likely that you are lacking many of the basic building blocks to success. You may find it hard to have confidence, believe in yourself, connect to others, and do the things needed to build the life you wish to create. You will want to use the Aroma Freedom process to clear out the negative beliefs and experiences that are holding you back, whether it is through self-guided sessions, online Aroma Freedom guided courses, or with a Certified Aroma Freedom Practitioner.

Score: 17 - 25
Some building blocks are in place

If you fall into this group, you are on the right track and have a reasonable level of self-esteem and confidence, and the ability to give and receive help from others. To really level-up your results, try setting some big goals and then doing Aroma Freedom to clear out remaining beliefs and memories that may be stopping you from operating at the fullest of your potential. You have a good foundation, now let's make it great!

Score: 26 - 35
The sky's the limit!

You have a solid foundation upon which to build whatever dream you desire. You have good self-esteem, can take pride in your accomplishments, are able to work constructively with others, and have cleared up most of your issues from the past. For you, it will be interesting to see what comes up when you try Aroma Freedom. Many people find whole new layers of memories and thoughts that they were not aware of when they start doing the process. As you continue to grow in your abilities, you will find that new things are possible for you you had not previously dreamed of. Keep up the good work!

Key Chapter Takeaways

We discussed three sources of problems in human life, as well as how Aroma Freedom provides a solution:

1 - Looking in the wrong place for the answer.

Personally - Reading books, taking classes, and trying things that really aren't leading you towards the solution.

Professionally - Following a theory about human problems that doesn't address the client's particular situation.

2 - Getting lost in complexity.

Personally - Following your endless thoughts about past and future, which leaves you confused about where you really are and what you need.

Professionally - Trying to untangle the web of the client's problems by looking at their history, cognitions, behaviors and actions and applying your theory of change to them, which only makes things more complex and confusing.

3 - Trying to build a new building on a crumbling foundation.

Personally - Trying to solve your problems by adding what you think you need, such as a new job, relationship, or habit, without first dissolving the problems with your current situation.

Professionally - Asking your client to engage in new behaviors or habits without first dissolving the source of their resistance to change in the first place.

The Aroma Freedom protocols in the following chapters will address all of these issues, which is why it is a reliable method for quick and lasting change.

Chapter 5

―――――― ❧⊱✦⊰❧ ――――――

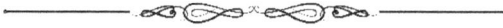

The Science of Aroma and Memory

In order to understand how and why Aroma Freedom gets results that are so deep, fast, and lasting, we need to first understand how the sense of smell is processed in the brain, and also how memory works. Once we have laid this foundation, we will be able to see how something so simple as smelling a specific essential oil, at the right time and with the right intention, can trigger a permanent shift in one's perceptions, thoughts, feelings, and memories.

The link between aroma and memory is easy to observe in your daily life. Smelling an apple can remind you of walks with your grandfather through the apple orchards back home. The smell of a specific cologne can remind you of an old boyfriend, with a surprising level of sensory detail. Memories that are evoked through the sense of smell tend to be richer in detail, more emotionally evocative, and take you back further in time than those evoked through sight, sound, or words. This fact has been clinically verified in multiple studies on what is called "autobiographical memory."

The sense of smell is closer, anatomically, to the emotion center of the brain than any of the other senses. The other senses (sight, sound, touch, taste) all route through the thalamus (the brain's primary sensory processing center) for brain processing before being routed to other parts of the brain. By contrast, the sense of smell is picked up by the olfactory nerve and goes directly to the amygdala (the brain's alarm center) first.

This is why the sense of smell can instantly trigger a feeling of disgust when smelling rotten food, or panic when smelling smoke. This "alarm" nature of smell is built into the brain for our survival. If you had to think about it very long before deciding whether to run out of a burning building, or whether to eat rotten food, you wouldn't live long enough to tell the tale.

The sense of smell is also involuntary - meaning, you don't have control over how you respond to a smell. In one study, Alzheimer's patients were asked to recall early memories either with or without being exposed to pleasant odors first. Those who were exposed to the odors pulled up memories that were more specific, emotional and real-feeling than those who did not smell the odor. This was not a function of whether they wanted to retrieve such memories - it happened automatically.

Aroma is very closely tied to memory in other important ways, too. The olfactory bulb projects to the amygdala, whose job is to determine whether the incoming sensory input is a warning of danger, or a signal to relax. How does it do this? By consulting memory.

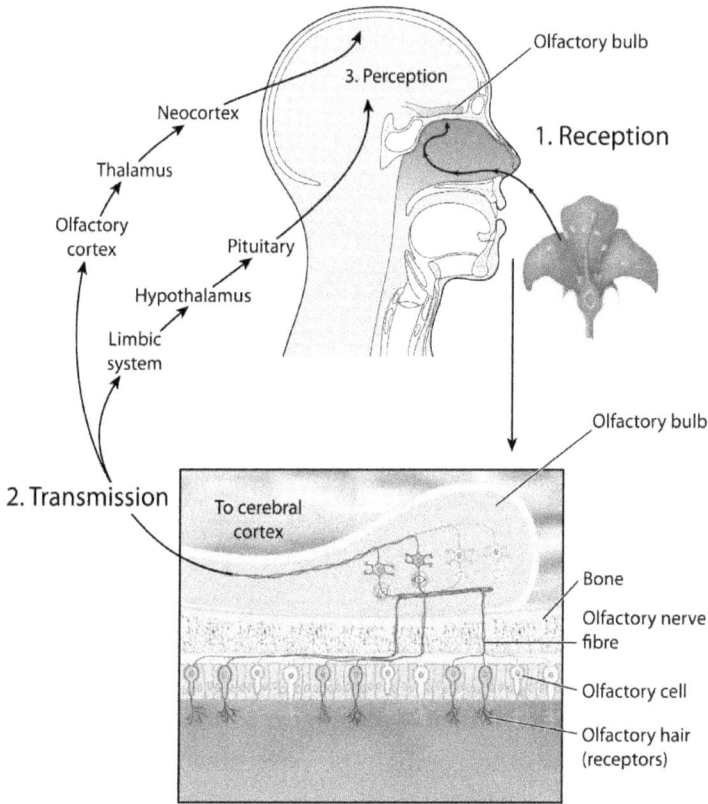

Next to the amygdala is another brain structure called the hippocampus. The hippocampus has the job of creating and accessing memories that are stored throughout the brain. So the amygdala sends a signal to the hippocampus, asking whether this sensory input is something that has ever been encountered before, and if so, whether it is dangerous.

THE LIMBIC SYSTEM

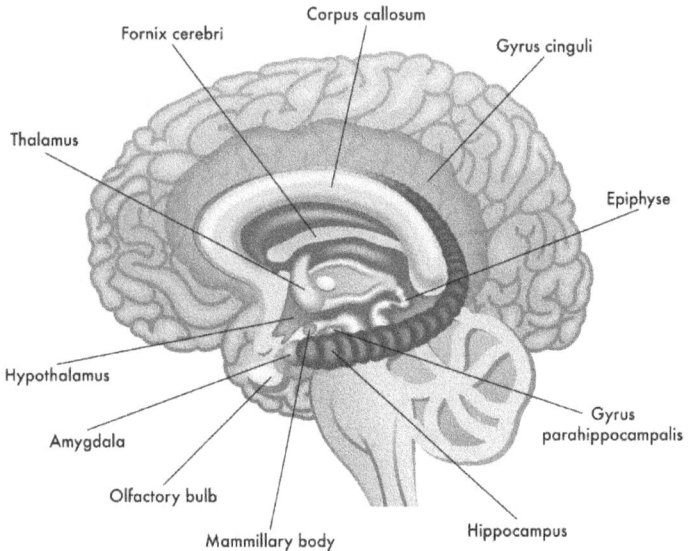

For instance, a rabbit encounters a fox in the field, it is chased, and it runs away to escape. The next time the rabbit sees or smells a fox, it will be able to run away more quickly. However, if it has been raised by humans and determines that they are safe, it will not run away. This is because its memory traces inform it that it is not in danger. All senses can be used as part of this triggering mechanism, but none work as quickly as the sense of smell.

In fact, "fear conditioning" is the term given to this phenomenon in the wild. Being able to learn what to fear and what is safe is one of the most primary ways that organisms survive. Interestingly, knowing "what to fear" can even be passed down genetically through generations. Researchers at

Emory University trained mice to be afraid of the scent of cherry blossoms by pairing the smell with an electric shock. The mice were allowed to mate and have offspring, and the scientists then found that their children and even their grandchildren were also afraid of the scent of cherry blossom, even though they had never been exposed to the electric shock! This shows that the memories consulted to determine what is safe, may not even be your own.

The important point here is that there may be scents that have been associated with wellbeing for millennia and the memories of this have been passed down through the generations, such that the smell of rotten food, toxic gasses, or a predator will instantly trigger a fear and protection response.

Conversely, when the sense of smell indicates that something is beneficial, the sense of peace and relaxation is triggered. This may happen when smelling a beautiful flower, delicious food, or a suitable mate. The smell of a rose, or lavender, or an orange blossom, will instantly translate into a sensation of delight and happiness.

We know that aroma affects memory, but how does it affect mental health in general? The most widely studied use of aroma in mental health involves the use of essential oils. Essential oils are tiny, volatile compounds that are usually distilled or pressed from plants. They exhibit potent effects in humans and animals due to both their aromatic effects as well as how they directly influence cells on a molecular level.

Generally, there are three main methods of essential oil

application, corresponding to three main schools of thought regarding how to best use them.

The "English" school of Aromatherapy involves application of essential oils on the skin. Traditionally in this approach, essential oils are blended with seed or nut oils (the carried oil) such as olive, jojoba, or other oil. This slows their absorption in order to prevent burning or skin irritation. Oils are often applied this way during a body massage.

The "German" school of Aromatherapy involves inhaling essential oils either directly from the bottle, on a piece of cloth, or from one's own hands, or else diffused in the air by a diffuser. This application relies primarily on the sense of smell, and works by triggering the release of hormones and other neuropeptides in the brain. This is the most common way that oils are used for emotional calming or balancing, and it is the method that we use in Aroma Freedom.

The "French" school of Aromatherapy involves ingestion of essential oils, either in a capsule, or with food or drink. This may sound strange to Americans, however in France, oils are routinely ingested for many health benefits, even in hospitals. In fact, the pharmaceutical product "Silexan" is actually just a capsule of Lavender Oil, and it has been studied to help anxiety as well as valium! In Aroma Freedom we will not be using oils this way, however.

How, exactly, do essential oils work in the brain to accomplish all of these things? There is still more work to do to gain a full understanding, but here is what we know so far. Essential oils are very complex compounds, and a single drop may contain up to 300 or more different types of active molecules. These work in synergy to accomplish things that the individual molecules cannot. Although the pharmaceutical industry regularly isolates specific compounds from essential oils in order to market them as a drug, they rarely work as well as the original oil with all of its complexity.

There are numerous studies demonstrating the successful use of essential oils for depression, anxiety, analgesia (pain relief), mood enhancement, dementia, Alzheimer's symptoms, memory, cognitive impairment, sleep, and more. If you are interested in the science and research behind essential oils, I will discuss this more fully in the Appendix of this book.

Meanwhile, here is a small sample of studies from labs around the world:

- Wang, et al. (2018) suggested that the anti-nociceptive (pain relieving), anxiolytic (anxiety reducing), and anticonvulsant effects of essential oils are accomplished by modulating the GABAergic system and the sodium ion channels in the brain.

- Ogata et al. (2020) showed that Lavender essential oil elevates mood by activating the central oxytocin neurons. Lehrner et al. (2005) showed a decline in anxiety, stress, and improved mood following inhalation of lavender oil.

- Chung et al. (2008) showed that the analgesic effects of

eugenol (a component of clove oil) occur through the inhibition of voltage-gated sodium and calcium channels. This relates to the ability of eugenol to potentiate the GABA receptors in a mechanism similar to benzodiazepines and barbiturates.

- Okano et al. (2019) showed that frankincense oil was able to reduce cortisol and stress markers in mice. Further, he demonstrated that the complete oil was more effective at this than when two of its isolated constituents, alpha-pinene and limonene, were administered separately.

- Costa et al. (2013) suggested that the anxiolytic (anti-anxiety) effects of lemongrass oil occurs due to its interaction with the GABAergic system.

- Jung et al. (2013) showed that Ylang Ylang essential oil was able to lower blood pressure and heart rate in healthy male subjects with just 60 minutes of ambient inhalation.

There are literally thousands of studies on essential oils and their effects on the mind and body. We know that they work in the brain in a way similar to some pharmaceutical compounds, albeit more gently. One of the main ways that essential oils have been studied relate to how they affect the opioid receptors (similar to anti-anxiety agents such as benzodiazepines like ativan, valium and xanax). Another has to do with ion channels in the brain that seem to alleviate depression and are affected by substances found in Frankincense oil. GABA (the main "calming" neurotransmitter) levels in the brain also seem to be targeted and affected by certain essential oils. In addition, there is an exciting line of research showing that essential oils can raise oxytocin levels significantly. Oxytocin is the brain chemical that is most highly associated with parent-child bonding, affiliative behavior, and approach behavior. In fact, scientists have found that lavender oil can increase trust behavior in research subjects compared to those who did not inhale lavender oil.

Additionally, we know that essential oils (in the form of resins and incense) have been used for thousands of years in religious and meditative practices. Burning frankincense resin in a catholic church, sandalwood incense in a buddhist temple, or olive leaves in an islamic mosque shows us how ubiquitous this practice is. There is an association between certain scents and generating the feeling of peaceful focus that is helpful for meditation and spiritual connection. Science has not yet caught up with the mechanisms of action for all of these practices, but there seems to be a connection between inhaling essential oils and the induction of specific brainwaves. Some essential oils have been shown to enhance alpha and theta brainwave activity, two frequencies that are known to be related to light and deep meditative states, respectively.

The question is not if essential oils work, but rather, how to use them effectively. The art and science of aromatherapy is itself vast, and people may study for years to become proficient in using essential oils for various mental and physical conditions.

This book limits itself to the use of essential oils for mental and emotional balance, and how to use essential oils strategically to dissolve negative thoughts, feelings and memories.

Luckily, you will not need to become a certified Aromatherapist in order to benefit from this book or from Aroma Freedom. I specifically designed the protocols you will learn in Part 2 of this book so that you can use a very small palette of essential oils to accomplish a great many benefits. We will discuss which essential oils tend to have which effects later. For now, just remember that essential oils are potent in their action within the brain, and that by using them in conjunction with the Aroma Freedom protocols, the results can be extraordinary.

Memory: Explicit and Implicit

Next, we need to gain a better understanding of memory and how it functions in our life. Usually when we think of memory, we think of a sort of movie or filmstrip we carry in our brains that is a record of everything that happened to us. When we remember something, we assume that we are accessing the original "impression" that the event made within our brain. We furthermore assume that the memory is eternal and unchanging - meaning that if we had a painful experience, the memory of that experience will always be painful. We think this way because that is how we usually experience it.

Upon closer examination, however, we see that memory is much more complex and interesting than that. For our purposes, we will look at two very different but related memory systems - Explicit and Implicit Memory

Explicit Memory refers to the memories that we consciously remember, such as events and activities, and is what we usually think of when referring to memory. It is the memory that we can talk about and refer to when telling stories, recalling math facts, or naming presidents.

Implicit Memory (or Procedural Memory) refers to the skills we have learned about how to navigate in the world based on our experiences, or the "lessons" we learned from those experiences. Implicit memory is usually not conscious - it is something we do, or act upon, rather than something we talk about.

An example of implicit or procedural memory would be learning how to type on a keyboard. Although we may have a conscious memory about when we learned to type (explicit memory), the memory of how to type itself is stored differently in the brain and works without our conscious knowledge (implicit memory). For instance, if I ask you to type your name on a keyboard without looking you could probably do it without a problem because that information is stored in your implicit, procedural memory, but if I ask you to tell me how all of the keys are arranged on that same keyboard you probably couldn't.

It is important to note that this classification system is based on the neurological observation that these memory systems use somewhat different parts of the brain. However, they relate to each other, and most memories involve both the explicit and implicit memory systems at the same time.

Some examples:

- **Explicit Memory (event):** Your uncle teaching you how to ride a bike.

- **Implicit Memory:** The physical coordination and inner sense of balance developed during that experience, that allows you to actually know how to ride. Also, feeling

- **Explicit Memory (event):** Getting mugged on a street corner.

- **Implicit Memory:** Learning that "I should freeze in fear when approached by a menacing person, do what they say, and I will escape alive."

You can see from these two very different examples that the "lessons" we learn from experience relate to both what we learn to do physically as well as how we learn to behave in order to navigate both threatening as well as non-threatening experiences.

The common thread here is that we are always learning about the world and about ourselves. From the moment we are born, we are busy developing a "map" of the world that includes experiences (what happened), but also conclusions we draw from those experiences, such as "I am smart but not coordinated," or "I can only get my way when I am stronger than everyone else," or "People only like me when I agree with them."

These conclusions we draw are, for the most part, implicit and unconscious, but they shape our responses in the world every day. If I have an implicit assumption that I can only get my way by force, then I will act in the world as a bully. I may never have consciously thought to myself "I am going to be a bully today," and I may even deny that I am being one because it was never a conscious choice. Nonetheless, it is the only way that I have learned to navigate through the world, so it is how I show up. At least, until this pattern is uncovered, examined and eventually overcome.

A memory, then, contains many aspects. It may include the explicit memory of the event itself. And it also may include the implicit memory of what we learned from that event, what conclusion we drew. In other words, what the event MEANT to us - what meaning we derived from it. This meaning could be positive, negative, neutral, or anywhere in-between.

Examples:

Positive meaning: I remember my uncle teaching me how to ride my bike. When I think about that memory I feel proud of myself, and also feel a sense of warmth and love for my uncle who showed me. This event helped me to become a confident person who feels loved and cared for.

Neutral meaning: I remember learning what the capital of Idaho was in 5th grade. When I think about it I don't really feel any emotional charge, positive or negative. This event does not really influence my future life that much.

Negative meaning: I remember the time I was scolded for

bragging about my perfect math score in second grade. When I think about it, I feel embarrassed and have the thought that if I show people that I am smart, I will get in trouble. This makes me want to hide my light and not shine too brightly. (This actually happened to me and did cause me problems until I recognized and cleared this memory.)

Now we can see the importance of memory for our current and future life-functioning. If we have memories that, when we think of them, carry a negative emotional charge, this means that they are carrying an implicit memory with a negative or life-depleting message.

The meaning that our past has for us, IS our roadmap to our future. Which brings us to one more very important distinction:

All memories contain an implicit **prediction** about the future.

In the last two decades, neuroscientists have been actively studying the role of prediction in brain functioning. The near-consensus now is that most of what the brain is doing on a daily basis is predicting how experience will show up for us. There are special brain circuits that are designed only to detect errors in our predictions.

When we toss a ball in the air, we predict that it will fall downwards. If it doesn't, then our alarm bells go off in our brain and we need to investigate what is happening.

When we are confident, we walk into a room and predict that people will welcome us.

When we are shy, we walk into a room and predict that people will ignore us or shun us.

Our memories are our predictions about what will happen in the future.

This leads us to the central argument of this entire book - namely that we can change our future by changing our past. In chapter 2, you saw dozens of stories of people who became liberated from the chains of their past.

Of course, we cannot change what happened in the objective past, but what if we can change what our memories mean to us? What if we can change the implicit learning we are deriving from our memories? Does that therefore change who we are in a very fundamental way? And, will that allow us to generate a future that is also fundamentally different from what we would have been had we remained chained to the past?

If I had never liberated myself from the memory of being in second grade and shining a little too brightly (and too obnoxiously), I would not have been able to write my first book that has changed countless lives, and I couldn't be writing this one. In processing that second grade memory I was able to make an adjustment - I could see that how I had expressed my pride in my intelligence was inappropriate and hurtful to others, and that is why I had gotten in trouble (and rightly so). But I could also update my implicit learning from that event. The 2nd grader developed a very simplistic implicit learning to just "not show others your intelligence." But this simple rule was hurting me later on when I wanted to write a book that would require me to use all the smarts I could muster. I needed to update that implicit knowledge to be something like: "Use all of your intelligence in the service of humanity. If you do that, you need not worry that it might hurt others."

Now what happens when we combine the power of essential oils to calm the brain and nervous system, with the power of memory as it influences our mood, emotions, and how we approach the future?

This will bring us into the heart and soul of Aroma Freedom. I created this technique to be right at the border between Aromatherapy and Psychology. From Aromatherapy we learn how potent essential oils can be to effect subtle and powerful changes in mind, body, and emotions. From Psychology we learn how reprocessing upsetting memories can create lasting changes in how we approach ourselves, others and the world. By combining the two, we gain an effect that is greater than each approach separately. We will go more into how this works in Part 2.

Key Chapter Takeaways

The sense of smell is your most primitive and survival based sense, triggering strong approach and avoidance behaviors.

Essential oils have been studied extensively for their effect on physical, emotional, and mental states.

Smell and memory are intricately connected for personal as well as survival reasons.

Explicit and implicit memories form the foundation of your understanding of yourself and the world.

You can use the power of essential oils and aroma to reprocess your outdated memories and create new neural pathways (to be described more fully in the later chapters).

A note about the Essential Oils used in Aroma Freedom

As you may have noticed, this book is about psychology, aroma, and memory. In this process, we use essential oils as the key that unlocks the memory complexes which have been keeping us stuck.

The specific essential oils that we use are described in greater detail in the Appendix at the end of the book. If you would like to experience the techniques described in these pages, please refer to the appendix to make sure you have the oils needed. In the Appendix, I also describe the rationale for the oils we use, where to get them, and how to make substitutions as needed.

Chapter 6

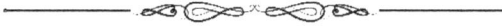

A Few Words of Warning

Before we launch fully into what Aroma Freedom actually consists of, how to do it, and how to understand the deeper mechanisms, I need to give you a few warnings. As a Psychologist for almost 25 years, and an essential oil user for 20 years, I have encountered some resistance to the methods I will be describing.

The primary resistance comes because Aromatherapy has gained a reputation as being too "wu-wu," "hippie," or only used in spas and salons for pampering delicate ladies and gentlemen who want to relax.

Granted, when we look at the mountain of research from around the world that supports the use of essential oils in clinical settings, it can allay those perceptions. Unfortunately, the average person is not aware of that research.

However, there is another problem we encounter when we want to use essential oils for true transformation. This comes from the fact that you can actually feel their effects! They smell good, they are relaxing, they are safe and non-toxic. The problem is that people use them for this purpose and then never go any further.

In the more everyday, casual forms of Aromatherapy, you simply smell an oil, apply it in a massage, or diffuse it, and feel the calming and relaxing effects. However, this effect generally lasts only as long as you are using the oil. If you make it a daily habit, you can have a daily effect. Many people do just this.

Here is the question: Why are you stressed or distressed in the first place? If you aren't able to dig in and determine this, you will always be, to some extent, chasing the symptoms of stress, depression, or anxiety.

I compare it with mowing the lawn. If you mow the lawn every day, you will keep everything looking pretty good. But you will never eliminate the weeds that keep popping up by just mowing the lawn. To eliminate the weeds, you will need to dig deeper and take the weeds out by the root. And this requires more than simply smelling an essential oil whenever you feel anxious, depressed, or upset.

I believe this is part of what has given Aromatherapy a reputation for being more of a superficial solution that cannot deal with the complex and deep problems that people struggle with regularly. And a casual, "smell oils to feel uplifted" approach is certainly not sophisticated enough to satisfy someone who comes to a therapist or coach for deeper transformation and life changes.

Don't get me wrong - putting an essential oil diffuser in a psychotherapy consulting room or a massage therapy or chiropractic office would definitely help create a nurturing and healing atmosphere and contribute to the overall effect of those therapies. But it would not be enough, by itself, to create the lasting change that is desired. Some practitioners may think that by simply letting clients smell a relaxing essential oil, they are removing the need for deeper work. However, doing this would be a superficial approach and would miss the opportunity for true transformation that I am presenting.

Another problem comes when people use low-quality or synthetic essential oils. The perfume and aroma industry is vulnerable to fraud and deceptive practices. This stems from the fact that high quality essential oils are very expensive to produce and distill. For instance, it takes up to 5000 lbs of Rose petals to produce just 1 pound of essential oils. Especially if they are grown organically, as they need to be, the work and care to produce this product is tremendous.

By contrast, synthetic compounds can be created in a laboratory very inexpensively that smell quite similar, and can be passed off as a pure essential oil to the untrained nose. Or, an odorless, colorless solvent can be mixed with an essential oil to dilute it and extend its volume 10X or even more without most people being able to tell the difference.

In fact, it has been said that France sells 10 times more Lavender oil than it grows! How is that possible? Only because of dilution, adulteration, synthetic laboratory products, and sometimes outright deception.

The problem with synthetic or diluted oils is this: Synthetic or chemically diluted oils will not likely have the therapeutic effect desired, and what is worse, may actually be toxic to the brain and body. When someone smells an oil and it has no effect, they may conclude that "essential oils don't work." Or, when they get a chemical burn from touching a synthetic oil or a headache from inhaling one, they may conclude that this practice is dangerous and should never be done.

By contrast, when we use pure, therapeutic grade essential oils, they are very safe, gentle, well tolerated, and effective. **See the appendix for more guidance on how to find the proper essential oils to use with the Aroma Freedom processes.**

Another warning:

Over the years as I have trained psychotherapists, coaches, energy workers, healers, and aromatherapists in the Aroma Freedom process, there is another problem that I have observed. Many professionals who have reached some level of competency in their field love to learn new things. That is great, and that is how they got so good at what they do! However, they have a tendency to mix the Aroma Freedom processes in with what they already do before they have truly grasped the power of what Aroma Freedom can do on its own. They may be skilled at balancing energy in the body or moving the chi using qigong - so they think that doing this while their client is processing a memory with Aroma Freedom will make it more powerful. But this only confuses the process, and confuses the client. Now the client thinks that they need to become a qigong master in order to do Aroma Freedom, which is not true.

Or, they may be skilled in a particular psychotherapeutic

technique, such as integrating parts of the personality, and so they get into a dialogue with their clients at the beginning of an Aroma Freedom session about their "parts," and soon the client thinks that they need to understand all of their "parts" to do Aroma Freedom. Which is not true.

I encourage practitioners that come into our training program to "leave everything they know at the door" so that they can learn how to do Aroma Freedom properly. This includes learning how to troubleshoot when a session does not go as expected. Although the techniques are simple, there are some subtleties that do not appear until in the presence of an actual client. Sometimes clients will take longer than expected to process a memory, or they jump around from idea to idea, or memory to memory. In these cases the practitioner may be tempted to think that Aroma Freedom is not "working," and they will jump into another technique that they know. Instead, I encourage them to bring up these sessions in class so that they can learn how to handle these difficulties from within the Aroma Freedom frame itself. There is an art to guiding clients (and oneself) to the successful resolution of problems using Aroma Freedom that we will talk about soon.

Staying within the guidelines that I will discuss in part 2 of this book requires discipline. It requires you to understand and do each step fully before moving on to the next one. This is why we review the purpose behind each step of the process. Once you know what you are looking for, it is easy to stay focused and engaged in what you need to do every step of the way, and the results that happen feel very magical. Actually it is not magic at all - just the predictable outcome of reconsolidating negative memories with essential oils in the way that we teach.

So I encourage you to really study and practice the steps until you have experienced the results you are looking for - whether this is for yourself or a client. Once you see the results, you will be hooked!

One final warning:

If you find yourself doubting whether this process can be effective because it is so simple, remember what I said earlier - **The technique is simple, but people are complicated!** Just because your problems feel overwhelming, frustrating, deep-seated, impossible to overcome, etc., does not mean that the solution to them needs to be complicated. When people wonder at how fast the results are, I remind them that changing one's perspective only takes a moment.

To prove this, let's try an experiment. Turn your head and look to the left. Take in what you see. Now, move your head to the right. What do you see now? Is the view totally different? Is there even a single thing in your line of vision that was there just a moment before? No! When you shift your perspective, everything looks different. And it only takes a moment.

Similarly, in life, we suffer mostly because our perspective shows us problems that seem impossible to overcome. But once we gain a new perspective, new possibilities emerge immediately.

Because the techniques are simple, there is a tendency NOT to do them when we need them the most. I will teach you a simple process in part 2 called the Aroma Reset, that only takes a few minutes, but can completely shift your emotions and attitude about problematic areas of your life. The problem is, it only works if you remember to DO it when you need it. I will give some tips on how to integrate these techniques into your everyday life in part 3.

Also, every Aroma Freedom session has an element of surprise. This is because we are accessing memories that you may not have any idea are connected with the issues at hand. We tend to search for memories based on context. That is, if you are struggling with a business problem, you tend to think that the source of your problem will probably be another time when you struggled with business. Almost always, however, this is not the case. In Aroma Freedom, we connect memories based on feeling. This means that your business problem may actually be related to a memory from 4th grade when you were not picked for the kickball team you wanted. Totally different context, but same feeling. Prior to your Aroma Freedom session, you assume you know what is causing your problem and that it is not fixable. Once the Aroma Freedom process reveals the hidden real cause of the problem, and then dissolves or reconsolidates the memory, the current problem itself appears totally different or even totally disappears.

So, do your best not to prejudge what Aroma Freedom can and cannot help. Instead, give it a try whenever you are suffering or want to boost your results, productivity, happiness, and freedom. It can't hurt, and might just be life changing. Give it a try!

Key Chapter Takeaways

A few warnings:

Aromatherapy can be relaxing or rejuvenating, but using oils without a step-by-step strategy will have more limited results.

Low quality or synthetic aromas will give lesser effects, or could even cause toxicity or injury.

Practitioners who already have therapeutic skills may be tempted to fold Aroma Freedom techniques into their existing framework too early, and miss the true power of these techniques.

Don't dismiss these techniques just because they are simple - remember that changing your perspective can occur in an instant, even when your outlook has been very dark.

Part 2:
THE INNER WORKINGS
OF AROMA FREEDOM

Chapter 7

⸱⸱⸱⸙⸲⸲

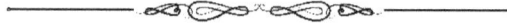

The Miracle of Memory Reconsolidation

(And How this will Change your Life)

"You don't get what you want in life. You get what you are."

- Dr. Wayne W. Dyer

The core feature of Aroma Freedom is based on the truth that, in order to reach a goal or go in a direction you want to go, you need to first go back and find the root of what is stopping you, pull that root out, and then move freely in the direction you are seeking. By contrast, if you persist against internally generated obstacles without resolving them, you will always be fighting against yourself and progress will be much harder.

We have learned that unresolved memories hold the key to what is holding you back. This is a truth first rediscovered in the modern era by Sigmund Freud, who found that many of his hysterical patients were actually suffering from Post-Traumatic Stress (although he did not use that term). He found that going

144

back and uncovering early traumatic events, and working them through in therapy, was the key to restoring his patients to good emotional health. His methods were revolutionary and have helped many people in the ensuing century-plus since he wrote of them, although now we use much greater precision in targeting and clearing memories light-years faster than he did (the average case of psychoanalysis is about 5-7 years). By contrast, people can change massively using Aroma Freedom and other techniques in a matter of weeks or months.

How has Aroma Freedom been able to get such amazing results for people all over the globe? What is the "mechanism of action" that drives its effectiveness? How is it we are able to "update our memories" in a much more positive direction so consistently?

When I was putting the technique together back in 2016, I had an intuitive understanding of why it worked, that went something like this:

When thinking of an emotionally charged memory, you have a certain **feeling**. This will probably be a stressful feeling like sad, angry, hopeless, powerless, etc. Then, when smelling the essential oil, this gives you a **different feeling** - usually something that would be described as "peaceful" or "relaxed." Remember, the oils are working powerfully in the brain on the opioid, GABA, and oxytocin receptors to induce the feeling of relaxation, even in the presence of an upsetting thought or memory.

At this point, your brain gets confused, because you are feeling two opposite things at the same time. Your brain then has to re-configure the belief about what the memory means.

For example, if your memory is of the time you were in a car accident and were trapped inside waiting to be set free by the firefighters, the feeling may have been one of terror. Every time you think of that memory you feel the terror in your throat. Now, when you are doing Aroma Freedom, this memory is activated and then you smell the essential oils, and suddenly you are feeling calm. Your brain has to negotiate these two viewpoints.

It is as if your brain is saying "I am remembering being trapped in the car, but I feel calm. Hmm. Maybe that memory isn't so terrifying now after all."

Spontaneously you get a thought that says "I am grateful I survived. I feel lots of love and gratitude towards the fireman who saved me. Maybe I will make a donation to the fire department."

What has happened is that the juxtaposition of two competing feelings has jarred the brain out of being stuck in the intensity of the original memory. As a result, you are able to make an assessment of the memory from the standpoint of being happy and relaxed now, and no longer trapped by the memory.[3]

---

[3] This, by the way, is the principal problem in PTSD (Post Traumatic Stress Disorder). Namely, that the person is "stuck" in the old memory, even to the point, during a flashback, that they cannot see present reality at all and are living entirely within the original, traumatic scene.

It turns out that Neuroscientists have a name for this phenomenon - it is called "Memory Reconsolidation." This is a process that has been studied since 2004 when a landmark paper showed that previously learned memories can be deeply "unlearned" such that the neural structure holding the learning in place is actually altered. In other words, the memory itself, including the implicit "what did I learn from this?" part of the memory, can undergo transformation to such a degree that a new neural structure is created.

Memory Reconsolidation can be accomplished in a number of ways, and we will review below how this occurs. We will also show how using essential oils to induce a new feeling at just the right time can greatly enhance and speed up the process.

This information puts us in a much better place to understand both **how** Aroma Freedom works, and **why** it works.

Memory Consolidation:

To explain how Memory Reconsolidation works, and how the sense of smell can enhance the process, we need to understand a little bit more about how memories themselves are formed.

When we experience something with at least a little bit of emotional intensity, we replay it in our mind over and over. Doing this "consolidates" the memory, and helps it move from short-term to long-term memory, where it can stay, potentially, forever. This process is called "consolidation."

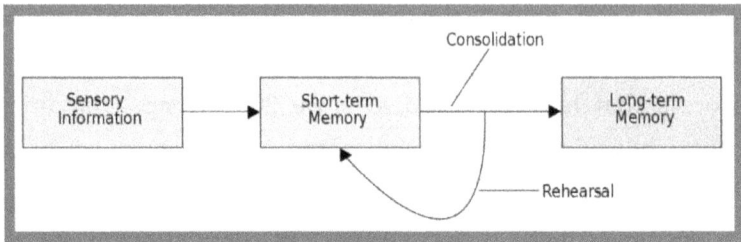

It had been the view of neuroscientists prior to 2004 that once a memory has "consolidated," it is forever etched into long term memory and cannot be altered.

For example, when a mouse is trained to become afraid every time a red light comes by giving it a small electric shock, the memory is consolidated through repeated pairings of the red light with the shock. Eventually, the mouse "learns" that a red light means a shock is about to come.

Explicit memory: "Red light and shocks occur together."

Implicit memory: "Whenever I see a red light, I should be afraid because it means I am about to get shocked."

This type of learning is very stable, meaning that even after a long period of time has elapsed, the mouse will still "know" that a red light means a shock is coming.

Now, if the mouse is exposed to numerous trials of a red light NOT followed by a shock, it will gradually reduce, but not totally eliminate, its fear response. This is called "extinction." It means that the mouse has updated its mental model such that now a red light means "possibly a shock is coming, but most likely not, but it still could happen."

In the laboratory it is observed that even after many trials of no shock following the red light, if you allow some time to elapse, and then show the red light, you can often observe some fear creeping back in. This means that the original learning of "red light = shock" has not totally been forgotten. It has been partially overwritten by a new learning, that states that the red light does not lead to a shock.

Now you have:

Old learning: "When I see a red light, I am going to get a shock."

New Learning: "When I see a red light, I am probably not going to get a shock."

Through repeated experiments across multiple species and multiple types of learning, scientists have confirmed the fact that learning such as this proceeds in layers. The early learning predicting that the red light leads to a shock gets covered over by the later learning predicting that the red light does not lead to a shock. Thus the animal carries on **for the most part** behaving as if red lights do not signal danger. Under certain circumstances, however, the fear will return. Even one exposure to red light=shock experience will re-trigger the full-blown fear response as if it had just been trained into them.

This finding is significant for phenomena such as PTSD (Post-Traumatic Stress Disorder).

A combat veteran comes home from the war and has learned to associate the sound of gunfire with danger. This is totally understandable, and even healthy given his experience. Back in his home country, he has to re-learn that loud sounds such as guns at the shooting range, or fireworks, or a car backfiring, do not necessarily indicate danger. It may take years of exposure to these non-threatening yet loud environments for him to learn that he is not in danger. Yet even in this case, it is very likely that a sudden, loud, unexpected sound will again trigger his stress response. The original learning of danger has been layered over by the learning of safety, but at any time, the original learning of danger can re-emerge.

This kind of "layering" of learning happens continually in everyday life as well, and gives rise to sayings such as "Once bitten, twice shy." Once we have learned something is dangerous, we will be cautious about it. This is a healthy response and is the basis of wisdom and understanding in life, and it is why older people tend to be more wise - they have had the benefit of decades of experience, during which they have been able to draw connections and learn what actions tend to lead to what types of outcomes.

Yet these kinds of learnings can also lead to problems and distortions that create suffering. When a child is abused, he or she may learn things like "Life is unsafe," "People cannot be trusted," "I deserve to be beaten," "No one is there for me," and so on. As mentioned earlier, the child is continually forming a map of the world and of themselves with each experience. The map may be life-supportive, filled with messages that bring confidence, hope, and strength. Or the map may be life-depleting, filled with messages that bring insecurity, anxiety, doubt, and pain.

Now we can apply the case of the mouse in the cage with the red light, to the case of a person who has grown up in an abusive environment.

Just as a mouse can eventually learn that the red light does not always mean danger, a child can grow to learn that the world is not always something to be frightened of. However, just like the mouse, the person is always vulnerable to being brought back to that scary place by something that triggers the original learning of fear.

This is why researchers, prior to 2004, were convinced that early learning was never fully replaced by later learning, and that the best we could do would be to keep strengthening our later learning of adaptive survival strategies. In other words, keep having experiences in which loud sounds are not dangerous, in order to strengthen the learning of safety. Keep having healthy relationships in order to strengthen the learning that people are loving. But, you could never actually erase the old learnings.

Until now…

Introducing Memory Reconsolidation

Memory Reconsolidation is a rather new concept which proposes that there are situations in which you can actually un-learn an original learning so completely that it will NEVER be triggered again.

This is a very radical concept.

Imagine if a combat veteran could un-learn the pattern of

responding to loud noises with intense stress, or an abuse survivor unlearning the pattern of fear of intimacy.

This is what is possible with Memory Reconsolidation.

Memory Reconsolidation is actually a process your brain does naturally, and frequently. Here is how it works in everyday life:

Let's say that when you drive down main street in your town, you see a car wash. Your friend is asking you where to get the car washed, so you tell him to go north on Main Street and he will see it in half a mile on the left. He calls you later and tells you that you were wrong, that it was actually on the right. You insist it is on the left, because that is how you remember it. You can visualize it in your mind on the left. Later, as you are driving north on Main Street, you realize that you were mistaken, and the car wash is actually on the right. You think, "That's odd…I thought it was on the left. I guess I was wrong."

What has happened here?

Your original memory was that it was on the left, and when you realized you were mistaken you needed to update your memory and put it on the right.

When you first saw the car wash, you had **consolidated** the memory incorrectly. As a consolidated memory, it had the feeling of truth to it - so much so, that you almost got into an argument with your friend about it. Now that you saw with your own eyes that you were wrong, you had no choice but to update your memory files. So you **reconsolidated** the memory.

It is a good thing that we are able to reconsolidate our memories. Otherwise, we would have no way of correcting information that was incorrect.

Scientists have found that Memory Reconsolidation has three distinct phases:

1. Activation of the memory.

2. Recognition of a mis-match between the memory and reality.

3. Updating the memory to reflect the new, more accurate information.

In the car wash example, the memory was first activated when discussing the car wash with your friend (Step 1). He tried to tell you that your memory was faulty, but you did not believe him. It was only when you saw it with your own eyes that you could see the mis-match (Step 2) and then update your memory (Step 3).

So now the question is, how can we update the emotionally charged and important memories from childhood and beyond, so that they can be a more accurate and useful guide in our lives? How can we help someone who has been traumatized, to recover from that trauma and embrace life without the memory of the trauma coloring every aspect of their life?

Bruce Ecker, Ph.D., in his groundbreaking book, <u>Unlocking the Emotional Brain: Eliminating Symptoms at their Roots</u>, explains that some psychotherapy methods lend themselves to Memory

Reconsolidation while others do not.

For instance, merely talking about a traumatic memory may help to some degree and bring some relief, but it will never achieve the kind of reconsolidation necessary for a full resolution of the problems that the memory can bring. For one thing, the memory needs to be activated (Step 1) - not just intellectually, but emotionally. The person needs to actually **feel** the emotion that the memory brings up in a visceral way. This is what someone with a traumatic memory tends **not** to do - the memory is painful, so they shy away from it.

Going further, even if the memory is activated, and the person is feeling the emotion viscerally, they need to accomplish Step 2 - Mismatch - in order for the reconsolidation process to continue. They need to be able to experience both the **feeling of the memory**, and at the same time, an awareness that the **memory is not accurate** in some way. When speaking with a friend or a therapist, the person may be discussing the memory and even their feelings about it, but what usually happens is the other person tries to comfort them by telling them that they are safe now, it wasn't their fault, and so on.

However, this is just intellectual knowledge to the person with the memory. No amount of telling them that they are safe will convince them that they are safe, unless they can **feel** safe **now, in the present moment**. How can a person be led to feel safe now? This can happen through several avenues, all of which involve some level of sensory engagement, such as:

- Awareness of breath

- Nurturing touch

- Eye contact and attunement by another person

- Gentle movement

- Soothing, gentle melodies or melodious voice

- Calming scents

- Etc.

This is called "bottom-up" processing, because it works from the level of bodily awareness to "reset" the emotional tone.

Once a mis-match is detected (Step 2), the person must now have a new experience for a period of time in order to reconsolidate the information anew (Step 3). In the case of the car wash, they had to see it with their own eyes long enough to be convinced that it truly is where they now see it to be. In the case of someone recovering from trauma, they need to have the new experience of safety in the presence of the memory trace long enough for the memory to truly shift into a new structure.

Memory Reconsolidation is a physiological phenomenon that happens at the level of the neural networks holding the memories in question. Here is how it works:

When a memory is originally created, or consolidated, neurons are coupled together in a network, just like wires are tied together in an electrical circuit. This is based on the concept coined by Donald Hebb, that "Neurons that fire together, wire together." Neurons fire together repeatedly, when, for instance, we mull over an event we have experienced until it becomes consolidated into a memory. Changes in the space between the neurons occur such that the memory becomes "durable."

Each time a memory is retrieved, the neural network is activated. Here is where it gets interesting. When a memory is activated and then there is conflicting information presented, the neurons actually "de-couple" and wait to see whether they need to be updated. Scientists have determined that there is a 5-hour window in which the neurons are "primed" to be re-written. If new information occurs during that time frame, the old memory is actually dissolved and a new memory is rewritten. Or at least, the parts of the memory that need to be updated are rewritten. If no new information is presented during the 5 hour window, then the old neural network is "re-locked" and the memory does not change.

This recipe for reconsolidation is the same no matter whether the species in question is a mouse, human, crab, or rat. If the organism has a nervous system and can learn something, then this principle applies.

Aroma Freedom accomplishes memory reconsolidation in the following manner:

Activation of the memory occurs by picturing it. It is made viscerally real by naming the feeling and finding that feeling in the body. It is further activated by identifying the negative thought related to the feeling.

Mismatch is achieved by smelling the essential oils. Because the scent of the oils creates a calm and pleasant feeling, this presents the brain with a "mismatch." The brain is expecting to feel a stressful feeling such as anger, fear, or sadness. When it suddenly feels calm and peaceful, the mismatch forces the neurons to "uncouple" and to become primed for reconsolidation.

Reconsolidation occurs as the person continues to breathe the oils into the memory. By having an experience of calmness while still thinking about the memory, the brain creates a new neural network that now includes the image of the memory joined with the more calm feeling. This generates new, positive meanings of the memory. Visually, the person may notice the image breaking apart, fading away, or simply losing its emotional charge.

This reconsolidation process is very quick, taking only minutes, and its effect is very noticeable and profound. Memories that just a minute ago seemed overwhelming, sad, or fearful, are suddenly seen in a new light. Sometimes this happens with just a single round of breathing the oil into the memory, or sometimes it requires returning to the memory multiple times and clearing the different layers of feeling that emerge. In either case, once the memory shifts, it looks and feels very different.

When a memory is reconsolidated, then the symptoms and problems that stem from that memory should change or disappear as well. For instance, if I was assaulted at a street corner and always felt my heart race when I walked in that area, this would be considered a problem related to that memory. If I were to have this memory reconsolidated, we would expect that the next time I walked by that street corner, my heart would not race and I would feel calm. Further, we would expect that I would not need to consciously try to remain calm, but it would happen by itself.

These are exactly the signs of true reconsolidation, according to Ecker:

"The true disappearance from memory of a learning that previously generated behavioral responses has the following signature features:

- A specific emotional reaction abruptly can no longer be reactivated by cues and triggers that formerly did so or by other stressful situations.

- Symptoms of behavior, emotion, somatics, or thought that were expressions of that emotional reaction also disappear permanently.

- Non-recurrence of the emotional reaction and

symptoms continues effortlessly and without counteractive or preventive measures of any kind." (Ecker, et. al. 2012)

Memory Reconsolidation makes personal transformation possible because it literally rewrites the neural network holding the thoughts, beliefs, and memories that give rise to many of the problems and symptoms that we struggle with. Once rewritten, the memories no longer trouble us, and instead can become a source of peace, wisdom, and inspiration.

In summary, Aroma Freedom generates true transformational change for people by helping to identify and reconsolidate the troubling memories that are at the root of many unwanted problems, symptoms, behaviors, and feelings people struggle with. It is a revolutionary approach that allows people to clear out years of emotional baggage and to gain access to the wisdom and inspiration that is available once they are no longer under the spell of negatively charged emotional patterns.

Key Chapter Takeaways

Memories are consolidated over time into stable representations of what you have learned about yourself and life.

Previous research assumed that new memories/learning were always layered on top of existing memories.

New research into "Memory Reconsolidation" shows that, under certain conditions, old memories can be "re-written" or even totally erased.

Memory Reconsolidation has profound implications for gaining freedom from problematic thought patterns, distressing memories, as well as the treatment of PTSD.

The Aroma Freedom process fulfills the requirements of Memory Reconsolidation by using the sense of smell strategically to rewrite old memories and their associated learnings.

Chapter 8

⸺⸺⸺⸺ ⦿⸙⦿⸙⦿ ⸺⸺⸺⸺

The Aroma Freedom Technique
(AFT)

Now we are finally in a position to discuss the Aroma Freedom Techniques themselves - what they are, how to do them, and what to expect from each one.

There are 6 Aroma Freedom Techniques, as delineated in the graphic below. They all use the principle of memory reconsolidation. They all rely on gathering 4 aspects of consciousness together - image, feeling, body, and thought - and then breathing specific essential oils into the image.

They differ primarily depending on whether the image in question is in the past (memory), the present (current life situation), or the future (imagined future situation). Some of the techniques take only a few minutes, whereas others may take 30 - 60 minutes, depending upon the number of triggering thoughts, feelings, and memories involved.

In the following chapters, I will first describe the two "long" techniques - Aroma Freedom Technique (AFT) and The Memory Reconsolidation Technique (TMRT). AFT is considered the "master technique," as it involves travel between past, present, and future, as well as goal setting, resolving memories, and creating future affirmations. TMRT, although a very simple technique, can be quite emotionally involved and sometimes taxing, as it often starts with memories that are traumatic or emotionally intense.

Then, in part 3, I will describe the four "quick" techniques - Aroma Reset, Aroma Boost, Aroma Wisdom, and Aroma Clear. These usually take between 1-20 minutes, depending on the context, and are designed for you to use "on the fly" at any time when you are feeling out of sorts - overwhelmed, frustrated, worried, triggered, etc. Although they are built on the same principles as the "long" techniques, they are quick because they may not be digging out the roots of your problems as thoroughly as the first two "long" techniques.

Here is a diagram describing all 6 techniques and how they interrelate:

AROMA FREEDOM

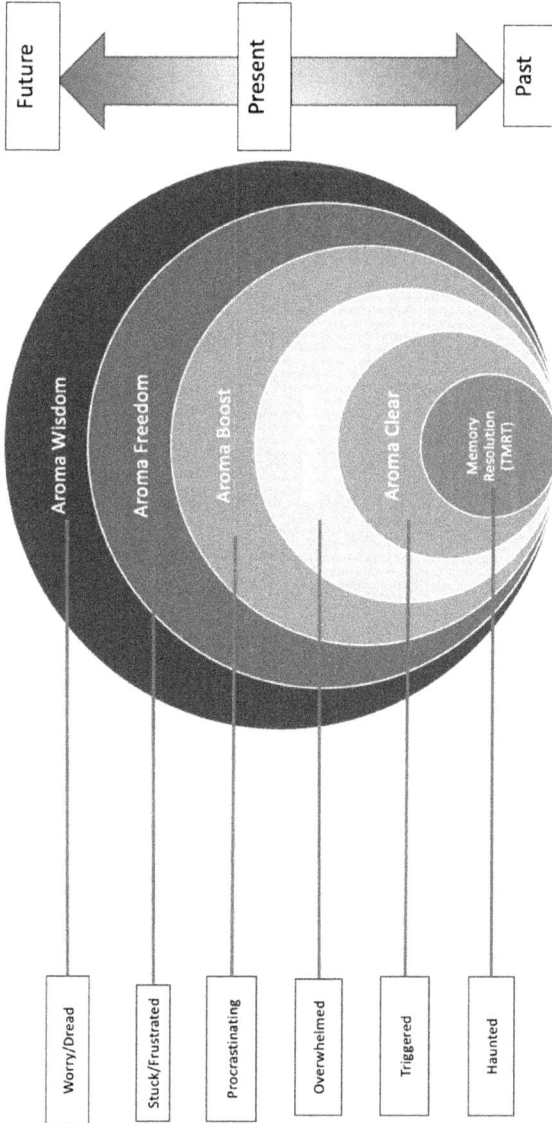

Future

Present

Past

Aroma Wisdom

Aroma Freedom

Aroma Boost

Aroma Clear

Memory Resolution (TMRT)

Worry/Dread

Stuck/Frustrated

Procrastinating

Overwhelmed

Triggered

Haunted

163

The Six Interlocking Techniques of Aroma Freedom

The Two "Long" Techniques - AFT and TMRT

The Aroma Freedom Technique (AFT) is a step by step process for identifying and releasing negative thoughts, feelings and memories that interfere with reaching goals and dreams. It is meant to be used to set a person's emotional energy flowing in a positive direction towards growth and expansion rather than contracting in fear, doubt and paralysis. It uses specific essential oils to trigger permanent shifts in how you view yourself and the world.

The Memory Resolution Technique (TMRT) is used to help you release a recurring memory, episode or encounter that you can't seem to feel better about. This technique can be used prior to an Aroma Freedom session if there is an upsetting memory that is not allowing you to set a goal or intention. Or, it may emerge spontaneously during an Aroma Freedom session. It may be a recent interaction or a long standing recurring memory.

The Four "Quick" Techniques - Aroma Reset, Aroma Boost, Aroma Wisdom and Aroma Clear (Covered more in Part 3 of this book)

The Aroma Reset Technique is a modification of the TMRT. This simple process is used to quickly reset your mood and emotions, giving you clarity, calm and focus in any given moment or situation. It helps you release the negative thoughts and feelings you have about a stressful situation. By focusing on your reactions and smelling specific essential oils, you "reset" your brain to return to feelings of peace and wholeness, allowing you to gain clarity on your next step.

The Aroma Boost Technique is an extension of the Aroma Reset. It consists of two Aroma Resets followed by a specific kind of affirmation. The new affirmation connects the next action step needed to progress the situation, the positive feeling you feel when you picture taking that action, and where you feel it in your body. It is designed to move us powerfully into positive action.

The Aroma Clear Technique is another modification of the Aroma Reset. It consists of an Aroma Reset but instead of breathing the oils into the current situation, we have the client connect with the feeling and drift back to an earlier time when they felt the same way. This often can bring up the deeper source of where the distress is coming from.

The Aroma Wisdom Technique is a variation of TMRT. But, rather than focusing on a distressing memory from the past, we focus on a distressing image of the future. This could either be a "doomsday scenario" of the world, or it could simply be a worry about something such as a child or personal finances. In either case, the image is processed just as a memory would be with TMRT until it is no longer distressing.

For all of the techniques, we use the same small palette of oils. These have been carefully chosen based on years of experience to provide exceptional results. See the Appendix for more information on the oils and how to get them. (If you do not yet have a Young Living Essential Oils account, contact us at www.aromafreedom.com/oils and we will help you get the oils you need):

- Clarity Blend

- Inspiration Blend

- Lavender

- Frankincense

- Stress Away Blend

- Trauma Life Blend

- Inner Child Blend

- Release Blend

- Transformation Blend

Now, let's go deeper into the two full techniques:

The Aroma Freedom Technique (AFT)

This is what we also refer to as the master technique. It goes the deepest, encompassing past, present and future. It helps us to identify exactly where we are stuck in the past, and opens us up to guidance for the future. It is the one you should use if you are not sure what to do. Here are the steps:

The Aroma Freedom Technique

<table>
<tr>
<td></td>
<td>

Step 1: Set Your Goal or Intention

Choose something you would love to see happen but are not sure how it could. Rate how likely it seems (0=Hopeless, 10=Totally Confident). Use Clarity or Inspiration oil if needed.

</td>
</tr>
<tr>
<td></td>
<td>

Step 2: Negative Voice

Listen for the negative voice that tells you this is not possible. Examples: "Yeah Right" - "You don't have the time" - "No one will listen to you" - "It will never happen"

</td>
</tr>
<tr>
<td></td>
<td>

Step 3: Feeling

Notice how you feel when you hear this voice. Make sure it is a **one-word** feeling or emotion. Examples: Sad, Angry, Overwhelmed, Hopeless, Frustrated, Afraid, Anxious, Embarrassed

</td>
</tr>
<tr>
<td></td>
<td>

Step 4: Bodily Sensation

Notice where you feel this feeling in your body. It could be in your head, chest, belly, or anywhere else. It could also be a bodily posture such as head down or shoulders slumped.

</td>
</tr>
</table>

	Step 5: Memory Connect with the feeling and bodily sensation. Drift back to an earlier time when you felt the same way. Notice the first memory or image that pops up, from recently or long ago. It could be a snapshot of a specific time, or a "movie" of multiple times.
	Step 6: Smell essential oils Put 1 drop each of Young Living Lavender, Stress Away, and Frankincense in your palms, and breathe the oils into the memory for about a minute, or until you notice the memory and/or feeling shift. For later rounds, use Inner Child, Release, or Trauma Life.
	Step 7: Notice what happens Observe what happens to the image, the feeling, the bodily sensation, and your thoughts. The image may fade away, break apart, become more intense, or shift into something else.
	Step 8: New Beliefs Notice any new beliefs, attitudes, guidance, or creative ideas that you become aware of. (This might not happen until later rounds.)

	Step 9: Rate your Progress Read or state your goal/intention again, and rate how possible the goal feels now (0-10). If there is still a negative voice, return to step 2. If there is no negative voice, move on to step 10.
	Step 10: Affirmation Create an affirmation that expresses your new, positive belief. This could be the same as your goal or a new awareness that you found during the session.
	Step 11: Power Pose Find a power pose that expresses the energy of this statement. Choose an affirmation oil such as Transformation or Believe. Smell the oil while saying your affirmation and standing in your power pose for up to 2 minutes or until the affirmation feels grounded and true.
	Step 12: Action Steps Make a plan and **take action daily**. Identify the next step or two needed to make your goal into a reality. Say your affirmation for 2 minutes morning and night for at least 3 days.

Tips: Repeat the affirmation in the power pose 1 hour after the session to make sure you are still on track. Record the affirmation into your phone and listen to it throughout the day.

Detailed instructions for each step:

Step 1 - Set your goal or intention, and rate how possible this feels:

AFT is the only one of the Aroma Freedom Techniques that start by setting a goal or intention. All of the others start with an existing concern, memory, or worry, and then process the emotional roots of that problem. By setting a goal, you are already beginning to move into a positive direction. When you set a goal, you activate the prefrontal cortex of the brain - the executive center. This already begins to pull some energy away from the limbic (emotional) system and starts the process of transformation.

Something interesting happens, however, when you set a goal. Whenever you make an intention to move in a new direction, your brain instantly begins calculating whether this will be possible. This happens automatically, and it is part of the process of accomplishing goals in life.

On a physical level, this could be as simple as jumping over a puddle. You see how big the puddle is, and calculate whether you can jump across it. A small puddle presents no barrier. A huge puddle, and your brain just says "don't even try." A medium size puddle, and your brain may ponder it for a little while. You gauge your level of energy that day, you scan your memory bank to remember times that you successfully jumped over something, and how that went. You also remember if there were any times that you jumped over a puddle and failed, ending up with wet feet.

If you are still in the game at this point and are seriously considering jumping, you will go even deeper - you will think things like:

- "Do I have slippery shoes on, and will I nail the landing or will I slip and fall?"

- "How deep is that puddle in case I end up in it?"

- "Is anyone watching in case I make a fool out of myself?"

Finally, you will make your decision to jump, or else choose an alternate action plan for getting where you want to go.

I bring all this up to show how every goal we set brings up these kinds of considerations.

For larger goals, the process is basically the same. Let's say you set a goal to grow your business by 50% this year. Your brain will instantly begin calculating the odds that this could happen. It will consider how successful you have been in the past, what obstacles you see before you now, and what opportunities and skills might help you.

In Step 1, after setting the goal, you rate how possible this seems at the moment, from 0=Impossible to 10=Totally Possible. This is an expression of your confidence that you can reach the goal. We will return to this rating after each "round" of clearing a memory, to see whether it is feeling more possible each time.

Most commonly, the rating will go up a couple of points in each round (i.e. - 2, 4, 6, 7, 10 or something similar). But sometimes a person will be stuck at a number for a couple of rounds (i.e. - 2, 2, 2, 5, 9). That is fine. Sometimes it takes several rounds to feel that a goal is more possible, even when clearing memories in each round. That is fine.

Sometimes, the number will go down before going up (i.e. - 4, 2, 6, 8, 10). That is also fine. In fact, when someone's number goes down, I congratulate them because it means that they are dipping into the deeper source of distress. It means that they will have a powerful clearing! Some of the best sessions progress this way.

Although we use the rating system as a guide, it is important to note that the GOAL of the session is not to get to a "10", the goal is to keep doing rounds of clearing until there is no more negative voice. Once there is nothing within you that tells you it cannot happen, the session can progress to the ending phase.

A note about GOALS:

Goal setting is an art and a science. The purpose of setting a goal is to give you a direction to work in so that you are not acting aimlessly. I personally am the happiest when I feel that I am moving towards a meaningful goal and can see that I am making progress.

In fact, here is my definition of happiness:

"You are climbing the hill that is yours to climb, and you feel strong enough for the journey."

This definition implies several things:

1. **You know what is "your hill" to climb.** You will never be happy if you are climbing a hill that is not well suited to your interests, skills, and inner calling. If you are pursuing a career that you chose just because it was expedient, or your parents wanted you to do it, or it was the only one available, it might not be the one for you. The hill needs to be **your** hill.

2. **The hill is not too steep.** If the hill you are climbing is impossible to climb, you will get frustrated and give up. That is not happiness. In this case you either need to find a different hill, or develop the strength and skills to climb the one you have chosen. All of these are acceptable options.

3. **The hill is not too flat.** If the hill is too flat, the journey will be too easy and you will get bored. You will not feel any satisfaction climbing it. It will not test you and make you grow as a person. In this case, again you need to find another hill, or you need to approach this hill in a way that makes it steeper, by, for instance, doing it faster or with more weight on your back.

4. **You feel strong enough for the journey.** This means that you have skills and resources that make the journey exciting rather than overwhelming and frustrating.

Of course the hill is just a metaphor for the journey of life, but my point is that there is a "sweet spot" in approaching life goals - when they are challenging but not impossible, and you feel invigorated pursuing them, then life is at its finest and you will have both the greatest satisfaction and the greatest results.

So when we start an Aroma Freedom session, we ask ourselves or our client:

"What is something that you would love to see happen in your life, but you are not sure if it can?"

There are two important parts to this question. The goal should be something you would love to see happen. It needs to come from your heart, and make you genuinely excited. Too often, we choose goals only because they seem possible, not because we actually want to do them. In Aroma Freedom we want you to choose a goal that is exciting and you are not sure if or how it can happen. Why do we insist on this? Because the sense of "impossibility" of a goal is usually rooted in past experiences and assumptions that might not be accurate. These past experiences are going to be reconsolidated during the Aroma Freedom session. When thinking of your goal, you will be finding all of the negative thoughts, memories and feelings that contribute to it seeming impossible. After those are cleared out, you will be in a much better position to determine whether the goal is actually possible, and/or what additional skills and strengths you will need to acquire in order to make it happen.

"End" goals vs. "Means" goals:

An "End" goal represents the end result you want to achieve. It is the actual life experience you are aiming for, such as "I live in a beachside house with my family, doing what I love." When you set an "End" goal and start the AFT process, you will hear all of the reasons why you don't think this is possible. After clearing those thoughts out, you will be in a better position to determine what you need to do to make this happen.

A "Means" goal is an intermediate goal that you will need to reach on the way to reaching your "End" goal. For instance, you may determine that you need to grow your passive income to $10,000/month in order to accomplish your "End" goal of living at the beach. In this case, you can set this "Means" goal and, again, clear out any doubts that you can reach the goal, and identify the steps you will need to take to make that happen. In that process, you will probably identify "sub" goals, such as developing specific skills and strategies for reaching each "Means" goal.

At each step along the process, you simply look at each step you need to take, and ask yourself whether you have what you need to be able to take inspired action towards that "sub" goal. If you feel confident and equipped for that task, then just go do it! If you do not feel equipped or if you have doubts, do an AFT session on the goal until you feel confident or have broken the task down even further to the point of making it manageable.

This is how I have used AFT in my life for the last 6 years, since discovering the process. At every step of my success journey, I just move forward with inspired action, or when I feel overwhelmed, frustrated, doubtful, or unsure, I do an AFT session on myself and get the clarity and confidence I need to move forward. This is why it is so important that you learn how to do AFT on yourself. When you have the ability to "clear" yourself out on a moment's notice, you can maintain momentum as you move towards your goals.

That being said, I also recommend that you have an "AFT Buddy" or a Certified Practitioner that you can turn to when you need someone to help you with a session when needed. Especially in the beginning of your AFT journey, or when feeling very lost, emotional, or overwhelmed, it is very helpful to have someone else walk you through the process. Even for myself, as the creator of the technique, it is helpful from time to time to have someone else take me through a session.

Step 2: Listen for the negative voice that tells you your goal cannot happen

As mentioned above, when we choose a goal, our brain will immediately begin to assess whether we can accomplish the goal. This assessment comes in the form of an "inner voice" that we can hear when we listen to it. This is "Step 2" of the AFT process. Say your goal, and then listen in. Take note of whatever you hear. It might say something to you like:

- "You can't do it."

- "You don't have the time."

- "You don't have the money."

- "You are not smart enough."

- "Yeah, right!"

- "That's a joke!"

- ...or something similar.

This negative voice is also called our "subconscious mind." It represents all of our inner "programming" about what is possible for us. If you don't hear a negative voice (some people don't), then just ask yourself how possible do you think the goal will be to accomplish.

Once you have accessed the negative inner voice or thought, just proceed to Step 3 of the AFT process. Don't judge it or argue with it.[4]

Step 3: Name the one-word feeling or emotion that you feel when you hear the negative voice.

This is one of the most critical steps in the process, and it is the one that separates Aroma Freedom from most other forms of casual conversation and even psychotherapy and coaching. The important point here is that we are not "engaging with" or "arguing with" the negative voice!

---

[4] After several rounds of AFT, you will say your goal and not hear any negative voice. Congratulations! Or, you may hear a positive voice instead, telling you something like "You can do this," or "Everything will work out fine." The positive voice may be a simple reassurance, it could be a word of scripture if you have a religious or spiritual background, or it might even be a creative idea. In any case, once there is no more negative voice, jump ahead to Step 10.

Many forms of cognitive therapy are devoted to trying to replace, reason with, or otherwise debunk the negative voice that emerges from our subconscious mind. When our friend tells us all of the reasons why she is not pretty enough or interesting enough to attract a relationship, it is our natural inclination to try to dissuade her from these negative thoughts. When she tears herself down, we try to build her up!

The same holds with most forms of self-help instructions. There are many books out there that instruct us to "argue" with the "Automatic Negative Thoughts" that emerge, to show them who's boss! We are instructed to counter those thoughts with positive thoughts. Now, this will work to some degree. When we replace the negative thoughts with positive, we might start to feel better temporarily. But there will always be the part of us that knows that we are just trying to fool ourselves. That is, until we can truly dissolve the negative thoughts and feelings, so that they literally are not influencing us any longer, as we do with Aroma Freedom.

Instead of arguing with the negative thoughts, or trying to interpret them or change them, we just ask one simple question: "How do you feel when you hear that voice (or thought)?"

It is important that we answer with just ONE WORD.

Why?

Because this ensures that we are not engaging with the negative voice, and that we are naming a feeling.

For instance, if the negative voice says "You are not good

enough," and I ask how you feel when you hear that voice, you cannot answer with "I feel like a failure" - because that is 5 words, not one.

It forces you to go below the level of your analytical mind, and to engage with the emotional/feeling part of your brain.

The feeling will become the key that will unlock deeper memories we need to access in order to clear out the negative thought.

Feelings vs. Judgments

In the Aroma Freedom Practitioner Certification Program, we spend a lot of time discussing the difference between Feelings and Judgments. This is a critical distinction that I first found in the work of Marshall Rosenberg, creator and author of the book "Nonviolent Communication."

In short, feelings are simple, one word descriptions of inner states, such as sad, angry, lonely, nervous, afraid.

Judgments are made when observing a person from the outside, without any empathy for the inner life of the individual. These would be statements such as "He is so lazy," "She is mean," or "I am a failure." You can see that they usually involve a comparison with an implied ideal or with another person. Also, you will notice that when you have one of these phrases applied to you, it does not feel very good. It is very common to judge others whom we don't understand, but it is also very common for us to judge ourselves. When we call ourselves a "failure," that is both a moral and a practical judgment, and all we can do is hang our heads in shame, or try to rally and fight against the judgment.

When you hear your inner voice calling you a failure, just ask…"What is the one-word feeling I have when I judge myself to be a failure?"

It may come up as something like "ashamed," "discouraged," "disappointed," or similar.

Interestingly, there is some strong evidence emerging that simply naming feelings already begins to change our mental state, and begins to reduce overwhelm. Lieberman et al. (2007), in an article entitled "**Putting feelings into words: affect labeling disrupts amygdala activity in response to affective stimuli,**" states the following:

> "Putting feelings into words (affect labeling) has long been thought to help manage negative emotional experiences; however, the mechanisms by which affect labeling produces this benefit remain largely unknown. Recent neuroimaging studies suggest a possible neurocognitive pathway for this process…The results indicated that affect labeling, relative to other forms of encoding, diminished the response of the amygdala and other limbic regions to negative emotional images. Additionally, affect labeling produced increased activity in a single brain region, right ventrolateral prefrontal cortex (RVLPFC)"

Lieberman is stating that when we label feelings (affect labeling), we reduce activity in the amygdala, and increase activity in sections of the prefrontal cortex (the executive center).

By naming a feeling, we begin to "get a handle on" the situation. We begin to understand what the situation "means" to us. For the purposes of Aroma Freedom, naming the feeling is how we access and dissolve the related memories. Once you have named the feeling in a single word, move to the next step.

Step 4: Find the feeling in your body

All emotions show up somewhere in your body. By drawing your awareness to the bodily sensations you feel in the presence of an emotion, this accomplishes several things:

1. It amplifies the feeling. Naming "sadness," for instance, and then feeling it "in your heart" only makes you feel it more. This is important, as you will remember that one of the requirements for Memory Reconsolidation is that the memory has to be recalled "vividly." It has to be "activated." Finding the feeling in the body is part of this "activation."

2. It confirms that you have actually named a feeling and not a judgment. There are some words that are ambiguous and depend on context to determine whether they are a feeling or a judgment. For instance, if you say "I feel weak," do you mean that you feel

physically weak as in "difficulty moving my body," or do you mean morally weak as in "unable to resist temptation." If you mean the physical feeling of weakness, you will identify it as, for instance, in the knees or legs, or all over the body. If you mean the judgment of weakness, you won't feel it anywhere as it is a thought, not a feeling. If you cannot find the named feeling in your body, go back and re-name the feeling until it is one you can feel in your body.[5]

This is usually a quick step. Once you have found the feeling in your body, move to the next step.

Step 5: Drift back to an earlier time when you felt the same way

This step represents the critical movement from "symptoms" to "root causes" that is so important for deep and transformative change from Aroma Freedom. When you drift back, you are following the feeling, and allowing yourself to notice the first memory or set of memories that come to mind. It is important at this stage not to prejudge what is emerging. Don't toss out the first memory that comes to mind just because it "seems" to be irrelevant to the problem at hand. In fact, it is important precisely **because** it seems irrelevant. Meaning, it has eluded your own attempts to solve the problem because it does not

---

[5] In this example, you would then say to yourself - "How do I feel when I judge myself to be weak?" The answer is usually one of the emotions you feel when you judge yourself, such as shame, guilt, disappointment, or it could be sadness or something else.

seem relevant.

For instance, let's imagine you are working on a business goal of making $10000 per month in passive income. Your process might look as follows:

Negative thought: "That's not possible."

Negative feeling: "Discouraged."

Bodily sensation: "Eyes downcast."

Earlier memory: "Trouble learning how to tie my shoes when I was 6 years old."

You might be tempted to discard this memory as irrelevant. What could such a memory have to do with making money as an adult? Actually, a lot! No matter what age we are, when we feel discouraged, we will have a tendency to doubt ourselves, feel less motivated, and give up more easily. And, if you have experienced this once in your life, you will be more likely to experience it again when a new situation comes up that "feels" the same.

So, make sure to go with the first memory that comes to mind. You will be amazed that, by processing the connected memory, you suddenly feel more empowered to deal with the current problem at hand.

Sometimes what comes to mind is not a single memory, but a whole sequence of memories that are related. You might picture all the times when you felt discouraged, or sadness, or anger, etc. In that case, I tell people to picture the memories "as if you were watching a movie, with the subtitle of "discouraged," or whatever the feeling is. Or, you may not picture a single memory, but rather, a specific time in your life when you had this problem. Again, just picture that entire time in your life as you breathe the oils in.

It is also important to note that, when working with a client, they do not need to tell you what the memory is. All that matters is that they can see the memory in their mind's eye. Not having the client reveal the memory can help in 2 ways:

1. Some of the memories that emerge are embarrassing, or feel shameful or uncomfortable to share with another person. By assuring the client that they do not need to share the memory, they are more likely to be honest and open with themselves and let themselves process the memory.

2. Some clients may want to tell their stories and engage with the practitioner about what happened in their lives. This is actually counter-productive in most cases. Once the memory has been accessed, we want to clear it out as quickly as possible, as that is what will bring them the greatest feeling of freedom in their life. There are exceptions to this rule - there can be times when discussing the memory will help them to process and integrate the changes they make. But in general, less talk is better when it comes to the memory.

Once the memory is pulled up, either a single event or a

"movie," we move to the next step.[6]

Step 6: Breathe Essential Oils into the Memory

Finally! After setting your goal, rating its possibility, listening for the negative voice, naming the feeling, finding it in your body, and drifting back to an earlier memory, you are now ready to begin smelling the essential oils.

As mentioned previously, we use a small but specific palette of oils to accomplish Memory Reconsolidation at this step in the process.

Simply drop 1-2 drops of essential oils on your palm, rub your hands together, cup your hands over your nose, and breathe the oils "into the memory."

For the first round, I recommend either Young Living Trauma Life Blend, or a combination of Lavender, Frankincense, and Stress Away Blend.

For the second round, I recommend Inner Child Blend.

---

[6] There are some people who just don't pull up any memory at all during this step. This could be for a variety of reasons. Some people are not very visual, and just don't process experiences that way. Or, their early memories are not accessible because they have repressed or suppressed the memories from that time in their lives. Or, for whatever reason, they are just "drawing a blank." In such cases, we don't let that stop us. Just work with whatever aspects you have available and breathe the oils into that. If there is no image, then just pay extra attention to the bodily sensation, and breathe the oils into the bodily sensation during step 6.

For the third round, I recommend Release Blend.

If more rounds are needed, it is fine to just circle back through the oils or choose any additional Young Living Essential Oils that you feel drawn to. Or, you may feel that at this point you already have enough oils on your hands that you can still smell them without adding additional oils.

Step 7: Notice what happens

As you breathe the oils into the memory, just notice what happens to the memory. Most people will notice the memory "breaking apart," "fading away," "getting less intense," or something similar. Sometimes nothing happens visually to the memory. Keep breathing into the memory using deep inhalations until something has happened.

You may feel the tension leaving your body, or the stress melting away.

You may find that a flood of new memories comes into your awareness.

You don't need to "do" anything as you are watching the memory dissolve. You don't need to "try" to make anything happen. It is important that you approach this process by just breathing into the memory and watching what happens.

It is possible that, as you breathe into the memory, your feelings will intensify. That is ok. If you are feeling sad, you may feel sadder. If you are feeling angry, you may feel angrier. When this happens, I always instruct people that "feelings are like waves, and no wave lasts forever." This instruction helps people to trust the process, knowing that, just as it is feeling the most intense, the wave is cresting and starting to recede.

And that is exactly what people experience. By just staying with the aroma (which is very soothing) and the breath, the memory processes and then breaks apart, recedes, or shifts into something else. For some people this happens after 10 seconds. For some it may take a couple of minutes. But it will happen. If nothing happens at all, we may need to troubleshoot the process (see tips section). Or, feel free to reach out to me directly at ben@aromafreedom.com with your questions and I will do my best to answer them.

To learn the process more thoroughly and experience it in a variety of applications, I encourage you to take one of our general interest classes, available at on the Aroma Freedom website - www.aromafreedom.com. We have classes on self love, prosperity, procrastination, and many more. Or, for a deeper dive, we cover all of this in greater detail in the Practitioner Certification, also available on the website.

Step 8: New Beliefs

This is sometimes called the "silent" step, because we don't always ask the client about their beliefs. In the first round of AFT, we usually skip this step unless the client spontaneously brings it up on their own. In the first round, the client may still be so deeply within their hopelessness or other negative feelings, that we don't want to ask them about new beliefs yet. It is premature for them to be focusing on new beliefs before they have begun really shifting out of the grip of negative emotions.

However, as they do begin to release the layers of negative feelings, it is almost inevitable that positive beliefs, attitudes, thoughts, inspired ideas, and creative visions will begin to spontaneously emerge. This is one of the wonders of this work - how the positive mindset emerges on its own once negative feelings have been stripped away. It gives one the sense that intuitive guidance, creativity, and positivity is our natural state, just waiting to be tapped into once the veil of heavy emotion has been released.

As the session progresses, I will, as a practitioner, begin to ask about the new beliefs that are emerging. I want to make sure that the client **notices** them. Especially when they come in the form of words of guidance, I want the client to verbalize these, as they will be very helpful in the final phase of the 12 step process, when we are forming an affirmation describing the new mindset that emerged.

If you are doing a session on yourself, pay attention to these words of affirmation and guidance you receive.

Remember when I was writing my first book, and I was unsure whether I could truly finish it within 15 days?

As I took myself through an AFT session and cleared away my doubts, I remember hearing a very clear voice saying - "A 150 page book? That is just 10 pages a day for 15 days…how hard is that??"

This inner guidance emerged once the negative feelings had

transformed.

But where did this voice come from? Was it my higher self? The Holy Spirit? My logical brain? Although it is impossible to say for certain where it comes from, we have learned that there seems to be a source of wisdom and guidance that each of us have the ability to tap into when we are not being tossed about on the stormy boat of reactive emotion.

In fact, it is my experience that we are **most** able to hear this guidance right after we have cleared away one of our big hurdles. It is almost as if the universe wants to reward us for going through the healing process by dropping a big, fat clue in our lap about what to do next.

An example of this phenomenon: One day about 23 years ago, I had a powerful emotional release session with a therapist (this was in my pre-AFT days). I had just finished releasing some emotion about my mother - something about needing her to "get off my back." After that big release, my therapist (wisely) asked me "What do you want now?" I don't know where the words came from, but I found myself saying "I want a spiritual playmate."

About 3 weeks later, I met my wife. And that is exactly what we have been for each other through over 20 years of marriage! It seemed that doing the emotional clearing somehow created the opening for a new level of clarity to come through. I don't know why this is the case, but you will observe the exact same thing with Aroma Freedom - after releasing painful emotions, you will have the most delightful clarity about how to stay on your best path going forward.

Step 9: Rate your Progress

After you have completed a round of clearing a thought/feeling/memory, it is time to return to your original goal to see how far you have come. Simply read your goal again and ask: "How possible does this goal seem now?" and then rate it again from 0=totally hopeless to 10=totally confident.

As mentioned during Step 1, the number might go up, go down, or stay the same. Any of those options is totally fine. Remember, the goal is not to get to a 10 (although that happens frequently). The goal is to get to a place where, when you say your goal, you don't hear or feel anything within you that says it cannot happen. The negative voice disappears, either replaced by silence, or replaced by a positive voice, guidance, or creative inspiration.

Remember that each session is unique and if a rating remains low, such a 1-1-1-2-3, or if it jumps around, such as 3-8-5-3-9, this does not mean anything is wrong with the session or with the person. It just means that their journey is either slower or bumpier than average. Do not make a big deal of this in the session, and do not indicate to the client that there is anything wrong with jumping around. Just keep doing the process and tracking changes until the negative thoughts have disappeared.

After getting the rating for the round, always go back to the goal, and ask - "When you say your goal now, is there anything else that the negative voice is saying?"

If there is a negative voice, go back to step 2 (negative voice) and repeat the entire process.

If there is no negative voice, move forward to step 10 (affirmation).

Step 10: Affirmation

Now that you have cleared all of the negative thoughts, feelings, and memories that were triggered by your goal, it is a good idea to strengthen and stabilize the new, positive mindset you are in.

We do this by creating an affirmation that expresses this new mindset.

A good affirmation starts with "I" and is spoken in the present tense, as if the reality you are affirming has already occurred and is happening now.

Examples could be:

"I write 10 pages a day."

"I am free to express myself."

"I receive clarity daily on my highest purpose."

"I am graceful."

"I am beautiful."

And so on.

Affirmations should always be phrases that feel good to say, are uplifting, and move you forward in the direction you would like to be heading.

Later in the book we will discuss some additional types of affirmations and even questions you can say at the end of a session to keep moving forward and to stimulate your creative mind.

Step 11: Affirmation with Power Pose

Once you have settled on an affirmation that captures your new positive attitude and any wisdom that has emerged during the session, it is time to select a "power pose" that will help to anchor the affirmation in your body as you say it.

Power Poses gained popularity following a famous "TED" talk given by Amy Cuddy from Harvard several years ago. Dr. Cuddy had studied how people who stood in power poses for just two minutes had more confidence and performed better in interviews, etc. than those who had not. In the original "Aroma Freedom Technique" book, I recommended integrating affirmations with essential oils and power poses during step 11.

In the book, I recommended two basic power poses, following Dr. Cuddy - the "superman" (arms up in victory) and the "wonder woman" (hands on hips).

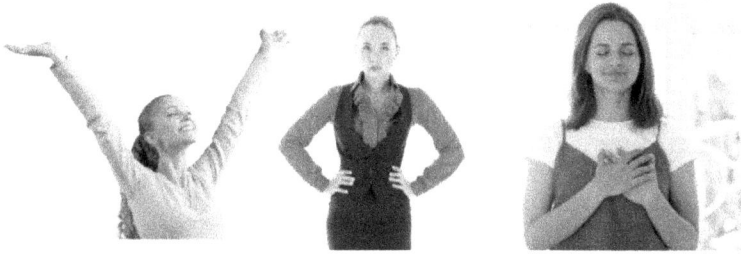

During the past 6 years of experimenting with and refining Aroma Freedom, we have added a third pose that captures more of an inward focus. We call it the "self-nurturing pose," and is simply placing the hands on the heart.

Once you have selected your affirmation, simply try saying the affirmation in each of these three basic poses. Find the pose that feels the best with the affirmation - that matches the energy of the affirmation.

Do not feel that you need to remain limited to these three poses - they are just good starting points. You could also choose a "warrior" pose from yoga if that speaks to you, or a prayer posture, or one with hands extended as if getting ready for a hug. I even had a client once who was a dance therapist, and she chose a "power dance" that she did while saying her affirmation. Have fun with it!

Finally, we like to combine the power pose and affirmation with smelling an empowering essential oil. The idea here is twofold: The essential oil adds to the exhilaration of the affirmation, and also by pairing the scent with the experience, it will strengthen the connection you have with your affirmation when you do it again over the next few days.

The oils I recommend for the Power Pose and Affirmation are either Young Living Transformation Blend, or Young Living Believe Blend. Transformation is more minty and uplifting, while Believe is more piney and grounding. Both are fabulous. If you don't have either of those, you can select any other oil that feels uplifting and empowering to you. Even simple lemon or orange oil can work well here. We are not as picky about the affirmation oil as we are about the memory processing oils because at this stage in the technique, we are more interested in simply amplifying the good feelings of the affirmation than we are in dissolving a memory (which is a bit more technical of a process).

Now, take a drop or two of your affirmation oil in your palms, rub them together, and smell them. Put your hands in your chosen power pose, and say your affirmation (preferably aloud if your environment allows it). Repeat the affirmation several times. Re-smell your hands and repeat the affirmation several more times in the power pose. Do this for a minute or two, or until the affirmation feels really true and real, and you feel uplifted and complete.

Step 12: Action steps

One final step before you end the session.

Now that you have named your goal, cleared your negative thoughts, feelings and memories, and said your affirmation in a power pose with oils, you have put yourself into a very positive mindset and are feeling confident that you can achieve your goal.

However, until you take action, most dreams just remain dreams.

For this step, focus on 1-2 action steps that you can take to begin to turn your dream into a reality.

Write down these action steps, decide when you will do them, and commit to them.

If time permits, you can actually sit down and plan your whole action plan for reaching your goal. However, this is often not practical to do right after the session, especially if a practitioner is working with a client. Unless you are a therapist or coach who specializes in helping clients identify and create action plans, this may not be something you feel confident or qualified to do.

Some coaches and therapists, however, do set this task up for the very next session. In other words, in one session they do an AFT session to set the goal and clear out the blocks. In the next session, they work with the client on their short and long term action plan. In the following session, they see how the plan is going and troubleshoot any problems in executing the plan. At any point moving forward, if the client is again expressing frustration, confusion, lack of clarity, or procrastination, they will immediately pull out one of the Aroma Freedom Techniques to clear out any of the obstacles that are emerging. Of course, if you are doing Aroma Freedom on yourself, the same applies: Use Aroma Freedom, create action plans, take action, and if you get stuck, do more Aroma Freedom to get unstuck for the next phase of the journey. In other words, rinse and repeat.

In the following sections, I will review the other Aroma Freedom Techniques. They are all variations on AFT, used at specific times when you don't need to do a full AFT session, or when it is more expedient to jump in with a variant. In our advanced Practitioner Certification training, we teach you how to actually jump around between the techniques during a single session in a way that amplifies the results you are able to achieve. This is discussed more in chapter 14 on Aroma Clear and Hybrid Sessions.

Key Chapter Takeaways

There are 6 Aroma Freedom Techniques, each used for a specific purpose:

Aroma Freedom Technique (AFT) - For releasing the thoughts, feelings, and memories interfering with reaching your goals.

The Memory Resolution Technique (TMRT) - For clearing traumatic or troubling memories.

Aroma Reset - For reducing stress and staying in the flow of life.

Aroma Boost - To overcome procrastination.

Aroma Wisdom - To transform fear or worry about the future.

Aroma Clear - To identify and release memories that are causing reactive emotions.

In this chapter, we also reviewed the 12-step AFT Process with tips for each step:

Step 1 - Set your goal or intention and rate (0-10) how possible it feels.

Step 2 - Listen for the negative voice that tells you it cannot happen.

Step 3 - Name the feeling you get when you hear that voice.

Step 4 - Find the feeling in your body.

Step 5 - Drift back to an earlier time when you felt the same way.

Step 6 - Breathe essential oils into the memory.

Step 7 - Notice what happens.

Step 8 - New mindset or guidance emerging

Step 9 - Rate your goal again. Return to step 2 if still a negative voice.

Step 10 - Create an affirmation that expresses your new mindset or belief.

Step 11 - Choose a power pose that expresses the energy of the affirmation and say the affirmation, in the power pose, several times while breathing essential oils.

Step 12 - Identify 1-2 action steps you can take that will progress you towards reaching that goal.

Chapter 9

The Memory Resolution
Technique (TMRT)

"The past has no power over the present moment."

— *Eckhart Tolle*

The Memory Resolution Technique

	Step 1: Identify the Memory Think of a memory that has a strong negative emotional charge. Once you can clearly picture it, go to the next step.
0-10	**Step 2: Rate the Emotional Charge** Rate how intense the feeling is, from 0=No Emotional Charge, to 10=Most Intense Possible.

	Step 3: Name the Feeling Find one word that describes how you feel when you picture the memory. Examples: sad, hopeless, lonely, fearful, etc.
	Step 4: Locate this feeling in your body Examples: Head, heart, belly, or anywhere else, or bodily posture such as feeling slumped over or teeth clenched. Once you have found it, go to the next step.
	Step 5: Identify the Negative Thought What is the negative thought connected to the feeling? Examples: "I am to blame" "I should not have gone there" "He will never love me"
	Step 6: Smell Essential Oils Place one drop each of Young Living Lavender, Frankincense, and Stress Away into your palms and rub together. Inhale deeply while focusing on the memory. Notice what happens to the picture of the memory, and to how you feel in your body and mind.

0-10	**Step 7: Rate emotional charge again** Think of the original memory again, and rate how intense it feels now. If the rating is greater than 2, return to step 3 above. Note the new feeling may be different. If rating is 2 or lower, move to step 8 below, or to "hybrid TMRT/ AFT".
	Step 8: Picture a happy childhood memory, or one that you wish were happy As you picture the memory, place one drop of "Inner Child" oil in your palms. Place one hand under your nose and one on your navel. Breathe oil into the memory for a minute.
	Step 9: Picture a strong image, like a mountain or tree Take a drop of Believe or Transformation Oil and breathe the oil into the image for a minute or two.

HYBRID TMRT/AFT

After step 7, you may skip steps 8 + 9, and move directly to a new Aroma Freedom Technique session. In that case, choose a goal that represents a completion or progression of the processed memory. This "hybrid" process is one of the most empowering sessions you can do and is highly recommended if you have the time and energy.

(OPTIONAL) AFFIRMATION

If desired, you may create an affirmation and power pose that expresses your new belief about yourself. Smell Believe or Transformation as you say your affirmation.

EMOTIONAL DETOX

Remember that you may experience fatigue or other flu-like symptoms for the next few days, depending on the severity of the memory released. If you feel out of sorts, you should drink lots of water, perhaps take an epsom salt bath, or do another Aroma Freedom or Aroma Reset Technique to get moving in a positive direction.

What is The Memory Resolution Technique?

The Memory Resolution Technique (TMRT) was actually the first technique I created, over a decade ago. It is a variant of EMDR (Eye Movement Desensitization and Reprocessing), a process I studied shortly after getting my Psychology License, over 20 years ago. I owe a debt of gratitude to Francine Shapiro,

Ph.D., the creator of EMDR, for her brilliant synthesis of depth psychology and solution focused methods into a simple treatment protocol. EMDR radically reshaped the landscape of trauma treatment by providing a much faster method of reprocessing traumatic memories than had existed previously. She also was committed to research, and worked for many years to organize and publish research studies showing EMDR's effectiveness as a treatment for PTSD (Post-Traumatic Stress Disorder) as for depression, anxiety, and more.

One of the results of this research is that trauma is now much more generally regarded as a critical piece to a client's overall treatment plan. There is now trauma-focused CBT (Cognitive Behavioral Therapy), trauma-sensitive addiction treatment, trauma sensitive residential treatment for children and adults, and more. People who have suffered severe traumas may require a different focus in their treatment plans from those who have not. When someone has had trauma, especially early in life, they may have more trouble forming healthy adult relationships, they may be more prone to addiction, chronic pain, focus issues, and more. Trauma affects every area of a person's life.

If you have suffered severe trauma and exhibit symptoms of PTSD, please seek the help of a qualified Mental Health Professional. Treatment of PTSD is beyond the scope of this introductory book. If you are already a Mental Health Professional, you will find Aroma Freedom to be an invaluable addition to the work you do. It will make your work faster, gentler, and more effective. You will need to take the Certification program to be able to fully integrate Aroma

Freedom into your practice. In the Certification program, we will discuss trauma and PTSD in greater detail.

For now, however, it is important for you to know that you can resolve traumatic memories from any time in your life, no matter how long ago. In fact, I want to take a moment to discuss the difference between trauma release and trauma resolution. When I wrote the first edition of The Aroma Freedom Technique book in 2016, TMRT stood for "Traumatic Memory Release Technique." This was to signify that memories that haunt you, terrify you, and weigh you down can be "released" so that they no longer bother you. By itself this is a huge benefit. To no longer be upset when thinking about an assault, war experience, rape, or tragic death of a loved one is nothing short of a miracle for those who have experienced it. However, this definition of what we are doing is not complete. When a traumatic memory is released, it means that you are not holding it any more, or more precisely, it does not have a hold on you.

But the goal in working with upsetting memories is not just to have them no longer bother you. Memory is how you think about yourself, how you construct your life and make sense of your life. You want to feel that your life makes sense, and that you are happy with the sense it makes.

I realized that what is really happening in TMRT is not so much that the memory is being "released," it is that it is being "resolved." So I kept the acronym but changed what it stands for - now it means "The Memory Resolution Technique."

Upsetting memories are incomplete memories. They refer you

back to a time when something bad happened, and if you still feel upset about it, then it means, by definition, that you are **still** not OK with what happened. In a sense, you have not **accepted** what had happened.

This is understandable. Many things that happen in life are painful, unwanted, disturbing, upsetting, and just plain awful. People may have been violent or abusive towards you, situations may have been unjust or unfair, losses may have been devastating. Who would want to accept that?

In a sense, every changing situation requires us to go through a mini grief process. We are all familiar with the standard phases of grief - Shock, Denial, Anger, Bargaining, Acceptance. Each thing that happens to us needs to move along that pathway somehow until we find acceptance. If we don't, then we have gotten stuck somewhere along the way. When we get stuck and can't accept what has happened, the memory will retain an "emotional charge" until we have gone back and completed the process.

The fact is, every situation we encounter requires us to respond emotionally to it. In the best case scenario, our emotional response helps the situation move towards a successful resolution.

For instance, let's say that you just learned that your college age daughter just told you she is not coming home for the holidays, but will instead be traveling in Europe with her boyfriend. How do you respond? Well, your initial emotional response could be sadness. This is the emotion connected with the awareness of loss. Now, do you show your sadness or do you hide it? If you hide it, your daughter assumes that you are ok with her plan and can go on her trip guilt-free. If you show it, perhaps she feels badly for ruining the family holiday, changes her mind, and decides to come home. In this case, showing your emotion served the function of notifying your daughter of the pain that her decision is bringing you. It prodded her to question her actions, and to make changes.

This is an example of how expressing an emotion (sadness) was able to move the situation along to a happy (for you) conclusion. In such a case, there will be no "residue," no "trauma" left over from that situation.

But we could easily imagine that situation moving in a hundred other ways.

For instance, let's say that when you first found out about your daughter's planned trip to Europe, you became angry instead of sad. Perhaps you yelled at her for being so "ungrateful." This set off a chain of unhappy insults which led to the two of you to both feel angry and hurt, and then stop speaking with each other. Now she is off in Europe and you are sad and lonely at Christmas.

To make this really tragic, let's imagine that 10 years go by and you are still not speaking. Every time you think back to that fateful conversation, you feel a jumble of feelings - angry that she has never come back and apologized, sad because you miss her, confused because you are not sure if you handled that situation the right way, hopeless because time is ticking and you are not sure if you will ever see her again.

This is a good example of an "unresolved" memory. Not only do you have strong emotion when you picture it, but the situation itself was never resolved - there is still an unresolved family rift that has never been healed.

If you were to come see me for an Aroma Freedom session, you can see that it does not really make any sense for us to "release" the emotions from that memory because it does nothing to resolve it, either in your own mind or in the real world.

Instead, a session might go something like this (Imagine an Aroma Freedom Practitioner is using the TMRT technique with you):

You: "I keep being haunted by this memory of the time when my daughter told me she wasn't coming home for Christmas. We ended up yelling at each other, and haven't talked since."

Practitioner: "When you think of that memory, how intense does it feel, from 0=no intensity to 10=worst possible feeling?"

You: "It is definitely a 10," you say, as tears start rolling down your cheek.

(Note: This is a good example of an event that was not "traumatic" in the classic sense like an assault, death, war, etc., but it is still a 10 in intensity because it represents something hugely painful - estrangement from a child).

Practitioner: "OK, name the feeling you get when you picture that event."

You: "I feel really guilty. I shouldn't have yelled like that."

Practitioner: "Where do you feel that guilt in your body?"

You: "I feel a clenching feeling in my chest, and my eyes are downcast."

Practitioner: "And what is the negative thought that attaches to that feeling?"

You: "I keep thinking that I was too harsh on her."

Practitioner: "OK, smell these oils."

You take a few minutes and breathe the essential oils into the memory. Nothing happens at first, but as you continue, you watch as the memory shifts. You see your daughter in the memory and feel a wave of sadness overcome you. You begin to cry more deeply, then as you keep breathing the oils, that subsides and you see you and your daughter hugging now in the memory.

Practitioner: "What do you notice?"

You: Explain what you just saw in your mind's eye, then say "I feel softer now. I don't feel guilty or angry any more. I just want to be with her."

Practitioner: " OK, so when you think of the memory now, how intense is it?"

You: "About a 5."

Practitioner: "And what is the 1-word feeling that you get now when you picture the memory?"

You: "Sad."

Practitioner: "Where do you feel that in your body?"

You: "In my heart and belly."

Practitioner "What is the negative thought that goes with that feeling?"

You: "I was always too hard on her. I wanted her to not make the same mistakes I did."

Practitioner: "OK. Breathe these oils into the memory now."

You take a couple more minutes and breathe the oils into the memory. As you do, other scenes from you and your daughter's life flash before your eyes. You recall yelling at her for getting a "C" on an English paper, and a few others. Then, as you keep breathing into this stream of memories, you remember your mother yelling at you and not understanding why she was so upset. You remember a time when you got in trouble when it wasn't your fault, and how you vowed at that time that you would never be like your mother.

Practitioner: "What do you notice now?"

You: "Wow. I just saw this whole stream of memories and I realized that I was doing the same thing my mother did to me. I need to tell my daughter I am sorry."

Practitioner: "When you think of the original memory of the phone call, how intense is it now?"

You: "0. There is no more emotional charge. I know what I need to do now."

We end the session after a little more discussion, and you have a newfound hope for the future. You are excited to reach out to your daughter and have a heart to heart. You also are thinking more about your relationship with your mother. She passed away several years ago, but you feel a softening in your feelings towards her and some empathy you have never felt before. You imagine there were probably reasons from her childhood as to why she was so harsh with you, but also have a strange sense that none of that really matters any more. All that matters now is just working to have the best relationship possible with those in your life now.

As hard as it may be to imagine, transformation really can be this easy.

Remember the steps of Memory Reconsolidation:

1. **Activate the memory.** You did this by picturing the memory while naming the feeling that was activated.

2. **Recognize the mismatch.** You did this by breathing the calming essential oils into the memory. Your brain was forced to recognize that there was more to the memory than your limited perspective. You began to see other

aspects of the situation. The neurons holding the memory now became labile, and ripe for reconsolidation.

3. **Update the memory.** The oils triggered your brain to scan your memory banks to find related memories, both in the life of your child, and when you were a child with your mother. As these scenes unfolded in your mind's eye, you kept breathing and noticing the new feelings emerging. Eventually, after several rounds, the original memory no longer had an emotional charge to it, and you felt clear and guided as to your next steps.

To review, we use TMRT whenever we have a memory that, when we think of it, we feel a negative emotional charge. This could be a "Traumatic" memory, or it could just be a memory that feels unresolved and incomplete.

Just follow the steps as outlined in the chart and you will do great! Note that there are some additional steps we can use once the memory has finished clearing. These are really just to support our emotions to move into a positive place if needed after processing trauma. They are not always necessary, but sometimes after resolving an intense experience, you may feel a little vulnerable and in need of comfort and strength. These steps provide that. We will talk a little more about the "Hybrid" sessions in part 3 of this book.

Key Chapter Takeaways

The Memory Resolution Technique is a simple and deep process for dissolving the negative emotional charge connected with a memory.

Memories that have a negative emotional charge are "unresolved" - which is why they can continue to affect you in the present.

You may have several layers of feelings emerge when you process a memory - such as fear, then sadness, then anger. Just work with the layers that emerge, without judgment.

Follow the steps and do several "rounds" of clearing until you no longer feel a strong emotional charge when you think of the memory.

Once an upsetting memory has been processed, end the session in one of several ways:

- Focus on a happy childhood memory and then a strong image as outlined in the steps.
- Create an affirmation that expresses the wisdom gained during the process.
- Do a full 12-Step AFT process, creating a goal that expresses a new direction that is now possible once the memory has been processed.

TMRT is not technically difficult, but can be emotionally difficult when painful memories are being brought up to be worked with. The memory does not have to be shared with the practitioner in order for the memory to be effectively processed.

Chapter 10

—————— ⚜ ——————

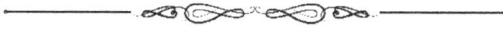

The 2 Keys to Making Aroma Freedom work for you

By now, you are getting the picture that we have the ability, through the Aroma Freedom Technique and The Memory Resolution Technique, to identify and release the negative emotional charge from memories that have been holding us back. This, by itself, is a huge breakthrough.

Previously, you would have had to talk to a therapist for months or years to slowly restructure your negative thoughts - and even then, you might still need to fight with your inner demons on a regular basis in order to maintain the freedom that you worked so hard to attain.

Or, you would work with a coach on getting the right mindset and tackling your challenges to become a better person, or more successful, etc. - only to find yourself repeating negative patterns because you did not have a way to release the emotional baggage you have been carrying with you into every situation.

The science of Memory Reconsolidation, as we use it within Aroma Freedom, shows us how to accomplish an incredible amount of healing in a very short time span. A process that might have taken months might now take just minutes! Memories that have been tormenting a person for decades might be gone or deeply transformed in just a few sessions.

This advance in your ability to transform your life so quickly creates amazing opportunities for growth - but it also may require you to re-think your approach to both your own life, and your approach to helping others, whether you do this professionally or not.

Because this approach is so quick and can so radically change your experience of yourself and life, I need to mention here two additional keys that will allow you to truly unlock your potential and to get the most out of Aroma Freedom.

These two keys are the **Spirit of Freedom** and developing a **Growth Mindset.**

Key #1 - The Spirit of Freedom

About 10 years ago, I was doing an exercise to refine my vision of the work I wanted to do. At that time, I was working in my private practice as a Clinical Psychologist, and I was also holding educational seminars on the benefits of essential oils and natural health practices to the general public. In this exercise, I was thinking about WHO I really love working with as a client or student. I remember that, when I posed this question to myself, I heard the statement **"I love working with people who want to be FREE."**

I realized that this captured a distinction I had observed in people over the years but had not made explicit until that moment. It seemed that some people came into my practice with a clear intention to grow, develop, and become the best versions of themselves. They needed help, of course (that is why they were there), but they were eager to do any homework I assigned to them, they were open and honest when doing emotional clearing work, and they made progress quickly. I probably attracted some of these people because they were referred by my other clients who had those qualities and I was known in my community as a therapist who was always doing cutting-edge stuff that appealed to these clients.

On the other side of the spectrum were clients who were pretty well convinced that their problems were all someone else's fault, which left them either hopeless or angry at the world. They wanted me to take away their "symptoms" (such as anxiety or depression), but had no interest in changing their lives or themselves in any deep way.

I know that therapists, like parents, aren't supposed to have favorites, but I couldn't help but enjoy working with the former group, and dread working with the latter group. Actually, dread is too strong of a word - In the beginning of my career, when I had fewer therapeutic tools at my disposal, it was easy to get pulled into the hopelessness of certain clients (these were the dreaded ones). But I quickly learned to take every dreaded client as a challenge - to discover where my blind spots were, and to learn new techniques and perspectives that could provide the needed breakthrough they desired. Over time, "dread" showed up less and less in my practice and was replaced by seeing my clients, even the challenging ones, as opportunities for growth (of my skills), and opportunities for breakthrough and liberation (for my clients). When someone came into a session hopeless and emerged confident and excited, it felt great for both of us!

The clients who had not yet discovered their journey of self-development but began to find their way and open up as they worked with me were particularly rewarding. I remember one client I worked with who had been raised in a strictly religious household. She came to see me due to some feelings of depression and hopelessness. During our work together, she realized that she had "settled" for an unrewarding marriage and career because she was just doing what she thought other people wanted her to do. As she recognized her own empowerment as well as her gifts and abilities, she made many life changes. Over the course of several years, she returned to college and launched a new career, started a new relationship and moved to a different city. I still get messages from her occasionally about how she is doing, and she tells me how much she has changed. She says that she can't believe how narrow her perspectives used to be, and how open she is now to everything life has to offer.

I don't have a good explanation for why some people seem to have this "spirit of freedom" while others do not. **I can define this "spirit of freedom" as the unwillingness to settle for anything less than a wonderful and rewarding life.**

To be clear, having a spirit of freedom does not mean that life will be easier - on the contrary, having this spirit means that when you are stuck in an unrewarding life situation, you **have** to do something about it. You refuse to stay stuck. You will take the sometimes more difficult road of facing problems head-on, searching for answers when there appears to be no hope, and always working to improve your skills and attitude so that you can transform your life for the better.

I have a saying I give to my students to help them understand this concept:

"Happiness is never guaranteed, but it is always possible."

- *Dr. Benjamin Perkus*

Here is what that saying means: There will inevitably be terrible things that happen in your life, such as the loss of a close family member, illness, pain, disappointment, betrayal, and more. When those things happen, of course you will not be happy. This is why happiness is not guaranteed - we can never sufficiently insulate ourselves from those types of events. However, when in the midst of any situation - **even a terrible one** - the possibility for happiness is always on the horizon. You may not see this possibility when in the middle of your suffering, when you are feeling pain, loss, despair, or hopelessness. But it remains a possibility. How do I know this? Because the human soul is infinite, and cannot be contained within the confines of any particular situation.

The famous Psychiatrist and Holocaust survivor Viktor Frankl demonstrated this when he was an inmate in a concentration camp in Nazi Germany. He wrote, in his classic <u>Man's Search</u>

<u>for Meaning</u>, that whenever he felt despair in the midst of horrific living conditions in the camp, he would picture his wife's lovely face and imagine reuniting with her. This would allow him to transcend the current situation until they could meet again. And, he noticed that among the other inmates, that the ones who had "something to live for" such as loved family members or a deep feeling of purpose, were the ones who were able to survive and not give up hope.

So, when horrible events occur in your life, or even just disappointing ones, or when you feel hopeless and stuck, it is important to allow yourself to feel the negative emotions coursing through you - such as sadness, anger, loneliness, etc. Don't try to pretend they are not there. Once you have felt the emotion, however, it is time to ask "What's next? What do I really want in this situation?"

In Part 3 of this book I will be showing you some quick techniques to help you quickly pull through the negative emotion and embrace the possibilities that are waiting for you on the other side.

In the meantime, here is a quick question to pop you into possibility thinking: **"What do I want instead of this?"**

Let's say that you are upset because you are bored at your job. You feel frustrated that the boss is not giving you opportunities for advancement, and hopeless about finding another job. It would be easy (and common) to just sit and stew on these feelings - developing resentment towards life, blaming the boss and maybe others, or even yourself, for your intractable situation. However this will not change anything.

When you ask yourself **"What do I want instead of this?"** something magical happens inside of you. Instead of focusing on the negative feelings and limited thoughts, you begin to imagine new possibilities. You imagine a world that does not yet exist, but perhaps could. On a biological level, you are shifting your brain state from the **limbic system** (emotion) to the **prefrontal cortex** (executive function, goal setting, future possibilities.) As far as we know, humans are the only creatures who possess the ability to really imagine a future and then set a course to make that future manifest.

Once you start living from this imagined future, everything changes. You can begin to strategize how to get there, you can take steps in that direction, you can start anticipating how good it will feel to reach this new reality. Your mood will lift and you will feel energized, motivated, and hopeful as you travel this path to the newly imagined future.

Of course, I don't mean to suggest that you will instantly feel better as soon as you identify how you wish things were. In fact, you may feel worse at first! When you compare where you are now to where you would like to be, it may even be depressing! But that is exactly where The Aroma Freedom Technique (AFT) comes in - you start by naming the goal, and then the technique will systematically strip away the layers of hopelessness surrounding achieving the goal, until at the end of the session you feel hopeful and confident that you can reach your goal.

In our previous example of being bored at work, you might decide that you want to have a new job in a different field altogether. Yet you feel hopeless about this due to feeling stuck in your current circumstance, not enough time or money to go back to school, etc. When you do the AFT process on this goal, you release these feelings of limitation and very likely will get an insight or idea about how to move forward. This idea will likely be unexpected and not something you had thought of before. It is still a mystery where these flashes of insight come from - some people describe it as the "Holy Spirit" speaking to them, for others it seems like the "Voice of Reason" or simply their intuition or inner wisdom. Furthermore, you can then take these inspired ideas and develop a step-by-step plan for implementing them. In our example, you may get a sudden idea for how to propose a new project to your boss that would excite you and not cost the company anything - or you may hear a quiet voice telling you that now is the time to quit your job and not to worry - that a new opportunity is waiting for you when you do. In either case, you have moved from feeling stuck/hopeless to feeling inspired/motivated.

Fancy Ninja Trick for transforming complainers into happy people:

When your client, friend, or family member is complaining about something, just ask them the question: **"What do you want instead of this?"** This question will pop them out of their complaining mind and into their imagination. Upon hearing this question, they will cease to complain about the problem and talk about what they want instead. This lightens the mood to begin with. Then, when they describe what they want, you can casually ask them how possible that feels, and what the negative voice inside their head is telling them about why it can't happen. From this point you can just follow the 12 Step AFT Process and go right in to clearing the negative feelings and memories that are making them feel so hopeless. Before you know it, your formerly complaining client (or friend!) is now hopeful and confident about their new future that they did not even know they wanted until they started complaining to you.

(Warning) - This might go really well. If so, great! However, if they look at you funny once they realize that you are doing something to them, just explain that you are learning a new technique for a training program you are in, and that it would really help you out if they could be a practice client. Most people will help a friend even when they won't help themselves.

In summary, the "Spirit of Freedom" is an attitude that inspires you or your clients to be the best version of yourself possible, and to work tirelessly to transform hopeless into hopeful, stuck into moving, impossible into possible, and settling-for-less into thriving-with-more. When you adopt this attitude there is a feeling of "unstoppable" in your pursuits. If you aspire to have this attitude but feel far away from it at the moment, don't worry - just keep using all of the Aroma Freedom techniques I am teaching you and this attitude will grow and strengthen. Every time you clear out a trauma, or a stuck-point in your mind or emotions, you gain the confidence that you can overcome anything. Even though there will be bumps in the road, pain, hurt, disappointment, heartbreak, deep loss, and tragedy in your life, these will not define you, but merely describe your journey. The moment you feel stuck is not the time to give up, it is the time to seek support through using an Aroma Freedom process on yourself or have someone give you a session to get clear and moving again.

Key #2 - Developing a Growth Mindset

Carol Dweck, Ph.D., in her groundbreaking book "Mindset: The New Psychology of Success," discusses a key distinction between two ways of processing information - two "mindsets." The question has to do with how one approaches success and failure.

When given a challenging task, a **"Fixed Mindset"** person will look at the task as a measure of his or her value or worth. "If I succeed, that means I am smart, competent, skilled, and a winner - if I fail, it means that I am stupid, incompetent, unskilled, and a loser." These traits are seen as inborn and unchanging, and those who have the good traits are just luckier than those who don't.

When given the same challenging task, the **"Growth Mindset"** person will look at the task as a way to learn something. "If I succeed, great! What did I learn? How did I grow? How could I do it even better, or differently next time? - If I fail, what did I learn? How do I need to grow? What skill was I missing that I could brush up on, so that next time I will succeed?"

Dr. Dweck found that this difference in mindset is one of the biggest predictors of success in life. Whereas everyone might admire Albert Einstein for his intelligence and accomplishments, a person with a fixed mindset might assume that he was just born intelligent and that is why he succeeded. On the other hand, a person with a growth mindset would understand that his intelligence would not have come to much if he had not devoted long hours to study, practice, experimentation, and of course plenty of failure, before finding the success for which he became so famous.

Since the publication of her book, which focused mostly on perception of one's intelligence being either fixed or free to change, researchers have come to realize that the fixed vs. growth mindset applies across nearly any domain of life.

For each of the following areas, here are some possible fixed and growth mindset attitudes (not an exhaustive list):

Domain	Fixed Mindset	Growth Mindset
Intelligence	I am only so smart, I need to only take challenges that I can understand.	I can learn and stretch my understanding, and I learn when I make mistakes.
Strength	I am a certain size and have specific limitations to my bodily capacity.	I can train my body to become stronger in almost any area.
Success	I have achieved a certain level of success and should not try to become more because I might fail.	My past success or failure is no indication of what is possible for me. Every failure is part of the path towards success.
Relationships	I can only attract a certain type of person and my relationships never work out.	I can learn new relationship and communication skills in order to find and keep a successful relationship.
Creativity	I am not a creative person so there is no point in pursuing any creative endeavors.	I can find a domain in which my creativity flows and I can cultivate and create more of it

		with practice.
Mental and Emotional Health	I "have" depression/anxiety/ etc. and this cannot ever change.	I can learn new skills and process emotions and trauma in order to be mentally and emotionally more fulfilled.

It is important to note that mindsets can be changed, cultivated, and learned. For instance, Dr. Dweck gives the example of children who were struggling in math. Half of the children were taught math as usual, and the other half were informed that their mathematical intelligence was something that would improve the more that they "stretched" their brains and tried challenging problems.

As you might imagine, the children who had been told that they could improve their mathematical intelligence did, in fact, improve more than the control group did. They were willing to try harder problems, and they were more resilient when they got a problem wrong. Rather than taking a failed math problem as "proof" that they were not good in math, they took it as a learning experience and as part of the larger journey of success - one that includes failure rather than being the "opposite" of failure.

These children were "taught" to have a growth mindset by simply giving them information about how the brain actually works. The principle of Neuroplasticity shows us that the brain will grow and change in response to stressors, repeated patterns, and being "stretched" by being asked to learn difficult things. Just knowing this information is very empowering - for those children, as well as for ourselves. When we know that we will be growing and changing in response to stressors and challenges, we are better able to embrace these challenges. Conversely, if we think that every failure is a sign that we are unworthy and doomed, we will tend to avoid situations that stretch us.

This is why having a **growth mindset** is critical for success with Aroma Freedom. For any given situation we encounter, having a growth mindset will empower us to see how much better we can make it. When we feel sad, or angry, or frustrated, or have the sense that "that's just the way things are," the growth mindset will allow us to wonder…"is that really the way things are? Or, can they be better?"

In the journey of success, there will be many points at which we feel stuck, confused, unable to move forward. We tend to look around, to look at our results, and to think that this is the best that things can get, because it is how things currently are. **In those moments, we tend to lose our perspective on what we want and focus only on what is.** Like the children learning math - those who thought their failure was an indication of how good or smart they were (fixed mindset), tended to stop pursuing learning hard problems. But for those who knew that the more they failed, the more they stretched and therefore the more they learned, their abilities slowly but surely improved.

When you learn the tools of Aroma Freedom, you become

aware that limitations are generally self-imposed, and that you will never know what is possible until you break down the restrictions you didn't know you had.

Here are some questions to pop you into a growth mindset so that you can consider your life from a new perspective and therefore generate new ideas.

- **"What do I want to change in my life?"**

  ○ This is the starting point for many Aroma Freedom sessions. By considering this, we can move into goal setting and the AFT process. Don't worry if it does not seem possible to change something. There is an old saying that I like, I am not sure where it came from: "Our job is WHAT, God's job is HOW." Just set the goal and let the process reveal the way forward.

I remember once I was doing a session with my daughter who was 16 at the time and who had just been dumped by a boyfriend. She was in the midst of her shock and sadness, so I asked her "What would you like to see happen?"

She answered honestly - "I want him to want to be with me again."

I resisted the temptation to tell her that it was beyond even my daddy powers to grant that wish.

However, I also knew that giving her one of MY goals, such as "Getting over the jerk and moving on" would not work either - because it was not HER goal. It is not what SHE wanted.

So, I suggested we do the session using her (unrealistic) goal as a starting point and just see what happens.

The session went something like this (shortened for clarity):

Father: "State your goal out loud."

Daughter: "I want him to want to be with me again."

Father: "How possible does that feel from 0-10"

Daughter: "0. He said he doesn't want to be with me."

Father: "Listen in - what does the negative voice say that tells you this cannot happen?"

Daughter: "That he doesn't want to be with me."

Father: "How do you feel when you hear that voice?"

Daughter: "Really Sad."

Father: "Where do you feel that sadness in your body?"

Daughter: "In my heart."

Father: "OK, now drift back to an earlier time when you felt this same sadness."

Daughter: "I picture us having that conversation."

Father: "OK, smell these essential oils and watch what happens."

I gave her a couple drops of Lavender, Frankincense, and Stress Away oils in her palm, and she smelled them, breathing them into the image of the break-up.

After about a minute, she looked at me and said that she got clarity that she doesn't really need him to want her, but rather, she needs to be aware of her own beauty and specialness. She immediately stopped crying, felt better, and went back inside to do some other things.

I was amazed at how quickly she shifted, and how on her own she got clarity about what she really needed and how to find it on the inside. I knew that if I just tried to TELL her those things, she would not have believed them. She needed to find them on the inside.

This is an example of an "unexpected" solution to what felt like an "intractable" problem. If I had had a fixed mindset, I would have been tempted to feel that there was nothing I could do - after all, I couldn't bring the boy back to her. But because I have seen the power of Aroma Freedom for so long, I knew that something could shift within her, even if I couldn't predict exactly how it would come about. In this case, I held the belief that she could **grow** through this experience and then used Aroma Freedom to bring it about.

- **"What do I think is fixed in my life that I am unhappy about?"**

  - There are so many aspects of life we accept, simply because we assume that there are not any alternatives.

By considering things we "think" are fixed, we open the door to consider changing them. (see example above as well).

- **"What is my identity and how does that limit me?"**

  o When we assume a role, we assume both the powers and the limitations of that role. Examples of roles could include husband, father, janitor, sister, daughter, brain surgeon, etc. We tend to identify ourselves by our role and then only act in accordance with what the role allows. By examining and perhaps changing the role we are identifying with, we can find new capacities we did not know were possible.

Example: Shortly after publishing The Aroma Freedom Technique book, I had the opportunity to again travel to Malaysia, Singapore, and Hong Kong to teach about Aroma Freedom. I had only recently figured out how to print books, sell them, and ship them within the US, but I was puzzled by the prospect of sending a few cases of books to Malaysia for the first leg of my international tour. I kept wondering about customs, taxes, fees, and I just did not feel confident that I could figure out how to do all of this.

Because I was unsure of how to proceed, I did an Aroma Freedom session on myself. As the session progressed, I realized that my identity as a Clinical Psychologist did not allow me to find a solution to an international shipping problem. At the end of the session, my affirmation was "I am a successful international businessman." I remember saying this affirmation, smelling the Transformation essential oil blend, and standing in a power pose. I noticed how differently I felt as compared to before I started the session.

Sure enough, right after the session, I had the idea to contact a printer in Malaysia who could print the books there and thus avoid the issue of shipping altogether. Within an hour, I had found a printer who could do the job!

By changing my identity to one more suited to the problem at hand, I was able to access the skills and abilities necessary to accomplish the goal.

Here are some other good questions for triggering the growth mindset:

- "What do I need to learn in order to reach this goal?"

- "What skills do I need to develop or practice in order to reach my goal?"

- "What failures am I afraid of experiencing?"

  ○ Your answer to this question will reveal a fixed mindset that you may not know that you have. Once you know where you are afraid of "failing" you can find a way to think about it as a learning opportunity instead.

Growth Mindset Questionnaire

Let's do a little exercise to help identify the degree to which you are operating within a fixed vs. growth mindset.

Below, rate yourself on a scale from 1 - 5 on how accurate the statements are—1 means "not accurate at all," and 5 means "most accurate."

Once you've rated yourself for each statement, total up your scores and then use the Answer Key to determine your next steps.

"Fixed vs Growth Mindset" Check-in Statement	Self Rating
I am convinced my life will get better through each new challenge I face.	
I see new and exciting possibilities for myself.	
I embrace failures as opportunities for growth.	
I welcome criticism of my work.	
I see my faults as areas for potential improvement.	
I don't mind "looking stupid" in front of others when trying new things.	

I would rather risk failure than play it safe.	
I see life as a continual opportunity for new discovery and growth.	
I view the problems in my relationships as exciting challenges to overcome rather than intractable dead-ends.	
When I don't know how to do something, I seek out new learning and mentoring.	
I work to improve my health and well-being by modifying my habits, routines, and lifestyle.	
I try new things frequently that I have no idea how to do, just for the experience of growth.	
TOTAL UP YOUR SCORE:	

What Your Score Really Means

Score: 12 - 24
You have a fixed mindset

If your score falls into this range, it is likely that you are stuck in a fixed mindset in most areas of your life. You may have experienced failures in the past that have convinced you that nothing can improve, and you feel nervous about venturing out and trying new things. You probably feel stuck in your life, whether it is in your career, relationships, or health, and you don't see how things can get any better. You may feel depressed about your possibilities in life, and anxious about where your life is going. Or, you may feel somewhat content in life but don't see it improving much in the future. You will definitely benefit from some Aroma Freedom sessions to open up to new possibilities that you have not been seeing. Try taking yourself through a full 12-step AFT session as outlined in chapter 6, or have someone take you through one if that seems easier. It is also possible that you are stuck in a fixed mindset due to trauma in your life that has trapped your nervous system in a cycle of fear and paralysis. By using the TMRT process discussed above and releasing these traumas, you will likely begin to automatically begin embracing more hope and possibility in your life.

Score: 25 - 43
You have the beginnings of a growth mindset

If you fall into this group, you are able to see new possibilities in at least some areas of your life. You can take some risks to grow, and the thought of "failure" does not completely crush you. You are able to take feedback and use it to make changes in your life. You can look at areas in which your life feels "stuck" and begin to find problem solving strategies to make improvements. However, there are still some areas in which you likely "pull back" or don't know how to proceed. You may be growing in some areas but stuck in others. With this score, I will recommend you take an honest inventory of your life and identify the areas in which you are feeling stuck or are assuming that there can be no improvement. Then, use this information to set new goals for yourself. Use AFT to find the confidence and wisdom to move forward, and re-affirm that every time you "fail" you are really just finding new ways to move towards success. Also, if there are traumatic memories connected with specific areas of life, such as failed relationships or business ventures, use TMRT to clear these so that you can get moving again.

Score: 44 - 60
You are solidly committed to a growth mindset

Congratulations, you (whether knowingly or not) have been adopting a growth mindset in most areas of your life! This may have come naturally to you, or you may have learned over time that no failure is final, and that you can learn something new and improve yourself in just about any situation. You likely enjoy taking on new challenges, seeking out learning and mentoring, and you regard life as a journey of discovery rather than a prison of fixed situations and abilities. For someone like you, Aroma Freedom will be an enjoyable tool you can use to accelerate your learning process, as you quickly find and release the stuck points you encounter as you are striving towards the attainment of your goals. Use the Aroma Reset Technique (next chapter) to stay in the creative flow as challenges come your way, or do the full 12-step AFT process to dig deep and release the remaining blocks that are stopping you from moving forward at full speed. Once you learn all of the Aroma Freedom techniques, you may find yourself drawn to helping others become free by giving them sessions either informally (family and friends) or professionally (becoming a certified practitioner).

Key Chapter Takeaways

The Aroma Freedom Techniques will set you free, but there are two keys that, when embraced, will supercharge your results:

The Spirit of Freedom is the mindset of wanting more out of life, being unwilling to settle for mediocrity, and being open to doing what it takes to find fulfillment. Some people seem to possess this quality more than others. Surround yourself with those people. When you feel hopeless, it means that you have temporarily blinded yourself to all of the amazing possibilities you are capable of. Keep relentlessly asking "What do I want?" until you get a vision, then use Aroma Freedom to clear out the perceived obstacles in your path.

A Growth vs. a Fixed Mindset relates to how you perceive failure. A growth mindset sees failure as an opportunity to learn from mistakes, grow, become better, and ultimately succeed. A fixed mindset sees failure as reflection of your worth as a human being, and steers you away from challenges so as to avoid looking stupid or feeling embarrassed, humiliated, and ashamed. When you embrace a growth mindset, you will see challenges and opportunities and become inspired by them. When you feel hopeless and stuck, it is likely you have slipped into a fixed mindset. Use Aroma Freedom to develop your growth mindset so that you can keep setting goals and expanding your capacities.

Part 3:
THE QUICK TECHNIQUES

Chapter 11

—————— ⚜ ——————

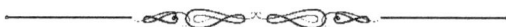

The Aroma Reset Technique: To Stay in the Flow

"The moment you change your perception, is the moment you rewrite the chemistry of your body."

– Dr. Bruce Lipton

So far in this book, we have discussed the history of Aroma Freedom, how it was created, who it is for, how it works, important keys to make it work better, and the two basic techniques (Aroma Freedom Technique or AFT, and The Memory Resolution Technique or TMRT).

You have learned about Memory Reconsolidation, which is the natural process by which the brain updates memories in order to integrate new learnings. I have shown you that we can leverage the power of essential oils and the sense of smell to help the brain to reconsolidate and update even the most traumatic, painful, or deeply entrenched memories and help a person find freedom and happiness beyond those traumas.

You have used the specific steps of the 12-step AFT process to find exactly which memories are holding you back and to release them so that they no longer exert a restraining influence on you reaching your goals. In this way, you have seen how shifting between past, present, and future allows you to free yourself from the chains of the past so that you can have a brighter future.

If you only use the two techniques we have already discussed, you will have a powerful arsenal for solving most of the emotional problems that come your way.

However, in this section, I will show you 4 additional techniques that will help you to get started QUICKLY to transform your everyday experience and to stay in the flow of growth, success, and accomplishment.

To review, the two full techniques we covered in the previous section included:

- The Aroma Freedom Technique (AFT)

- The Memory Resolution Technique (TMRT)

The four quick techniques we will cover in the next 4 chapters are:

- The Aroma Reset Technique - For staying in the flow

- The Aroma Boost Technique - For banishing procrastination

- The Aroma Wisdom Technique - For transforming

worry into wisdom

-   The Aroma Clear Technique - For releasing emotional triggers

Let's get started!

The Aroma Reset Technique

	Step 1: Identify the Situation Think of a current situation that feels overwhelming, frustrating or confusing. Once you can clearly picture it, go to the next step.
	Step 2: Name the Feeling Find one word that describes how you feel when you picture the situation. Examples: sad, hopeless, lonely, fearful, etc.
	Step 3: Locate this feeling in your body Examples: Head, heart, belly, or anywhere else, or bodily posture such as feeling slumped over or teeth clenched Once you have found it, go to the next step.

	Step 4: Identify the Negative Thought What is the negative thought connected to the feeling? Examples: "I don't have enough time" "I don't have enough money" "I am not smart enough"
	Step 5: Smell Essential Oils Place one drop each of Young Living Lavender, Frankincense, and Stress Away into your palms and rub together. Inhale deeply while focusing on the situation. Notice what happens to the picture of the situation, and to how you feel in your body and mind.
	Step 6: Decide what is next. If you are: A) Still agitated about the situation - Go back and clear another negative feeling related to this situation (step 1) B) Feeling calm - Get on with your day C) Realizing that there is a bigger issue you need to clear - Do a full Aroma Freedom Technique Session

The Aroma Reset Technique (or just Aroma Reset) is the simplest of all of the Aroma Freedom Techniques. It can take as little as one minute to do, once you learn and are comfortable with the steps.

To understand Aroma Reset, there is one additional concept that will be important to grasp. Take a look at this picture:

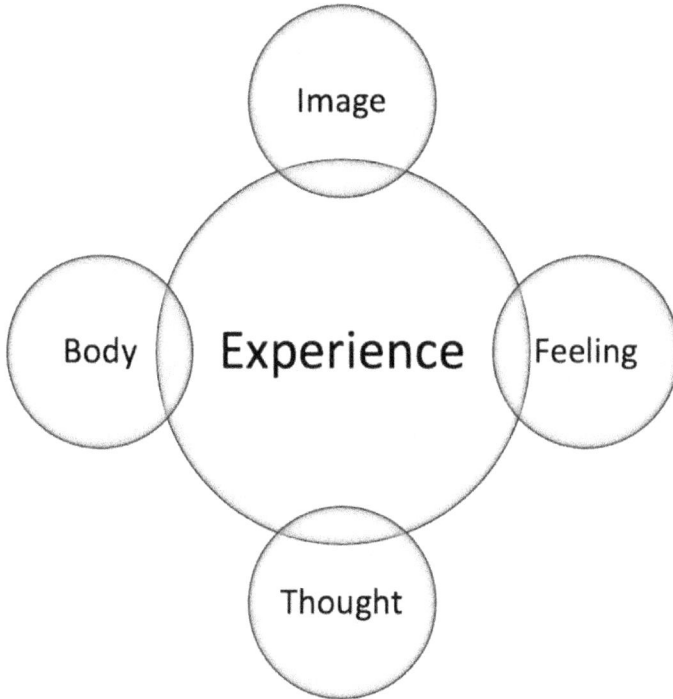

This model represents how experience is organized for human beings. As you will recall, The Memory Resolution Technique (TMRT) instructs you to pay attention to the image of the memory, the feeling you have when picturing it, the negative thought connected with the feeling, and the bodily sensations connected with the memory and the feeling. After pulling up these 4 aspects, processing can begin using essential oils.

With TMRT, the image is always a "past memory." Several years ago, however, I realized that the image did not need to be a "past memory," but it could refer to how you picture a present situation. When you picture a current situation in your life, it is likely that you are imagining **something** - whether it is someone's face, an image of a computer with tax software on it, your daughter, your messy house, etc. And, when you picture that situation, you likely have a feeling about it. This feeling is a measure of how well or how poorly the situation is going. If your business is going well and you picture it, you will feel something positive - like pride, happiness, satisfaction, contentment, etc. On the other hand, if your business is struggling, the same image will now bring you feelings of anxiety, worry, despair, frustration, or something similar.

Armed with this concept, we can now see how the Aroma Reset is structured. Rather than starting with a goal (as in AFT), or with an upsetting memory (as in TMRT), the Aroma Reset will start with a **current situation** that feels overwhelming, frustrating, confusing, or something similar. The specific instruction is to choose ONE situation in your life in which you feel this way. If you have ten upsetting situations you are dealing with, just choose ONE and do the reset on that. You can always go back and do another reset on the other situations later.

As per the instructions, once you have selected the situation, name the feeling, find it in your body, and connect the negative thought that goes with the feeling. You will note that this is exactly the same as what we are doing with TMRT, except it is a current, rather than a past, situation. Also, we do not bother to use a rating scale for the Aroma Reset, because we want to make the process as quick as possible.

As you breathe the essential oils into the situation, you will notice your body relaxing, and the feeling becoming lighter or dissolving altogether. After this has shifted as far as it is going to, check in to see how you are feeling now. Many times after just one round of clearing, you will feel refreshed and ready to face the day. If so, go do that!

About half of the time, a second round of clearing is needed. In that case, just return to the image of the original situation, and name the NEW feeling you get. The new feeling may be a lesser version of your original feeling. If your first round feeling was "Anxious," (more intense) then the second round might be "Nervous" (less intense). Or, the new feeling might be totally different from the original, such as moving from "Anxious" to "Angry." Either way is fine.

Usually after two rounds, you will feel refreshed and "reset."

Occasionally, however, a couple of other things may happen. You may have a memory spontaneously pop into your head, usually of an earlier time that felt similar. If this happens, just breathe the oils into the new memory and notice what occurs. After that memory processes, just return to the original situation and see how it feels. (NOTE: We will discuss this phenomenon more in the section on Aroma Clear.)

Or, you may realize, when processing the situation, that this is actually a bigger issue than you had first thought, and that you really need to do a full AFT or TMRT session on the issue. In either case, the Aroma Reset was helpful because it got you to the place of knowing what you need to do next.

Example:

I remember one time, shortly after I had discovered the Aroma Reset, we had a chance to try it out in our life. My wife and I were folding clothes in the bedroom, and our cat was on our bed. The cat began making some coughing sounds, and I knew this meant she was about to cough up a furball. Since I didn't want that mess on our comforter, I quickly reached over and grabbed the cat, and set her on the floor, where she proceeded to cough up the expected furball. I cleaned it up and we went about our day.

About 15 minutes later, though, I noticed that my wife seemed very agitated. She was short tempered and seemed to be on the verge of tears. I asked her what was going on. She said that, when I grabbed our cat and put her on the floor, she was shocked and worried that I was going to hurt the cat. Something about the suddenness of my movement had startled her into thinking this. I, of course, had no idea that this affected her so much, as I was never intending to hurt the cat.

I suggested that she do an Aroma Reset. I led her through the process by having her picture the situation - she was able to vividly pull up the image of me reaching quickly for the cat. She named the feeling of "fear" and could feel it in her belly. The negative thought was - "He's going to hurt her."

Once she had this pulled up, I gave her a drop or two of essential oils and had her breathe into that image. Sure enough, within about 30 seconds, her shoulders relaxed, and her fear went away. The image dissolved. She was able to realize **emotionally** what she already knew **intellectually** - that the cat was safe, and that her husband was not a cat-torturer.

More importantly, we were able to get on with our day. I imagine what would have happened if we had not done the reset that day. I had no idea that my wife had been triggered by anything. She herself may not have been able to verbalize exactly what was wrong. She just would have been in a sour mood, or agitated, or easily triggered. We might have gotten into a fight about something totally unrelated. This is what happens when people walk around with unresolved emotional reactions. We don't know why we are agitated, and end up taking out our emotions in the wrong places, just like a person frustrated at work might come home and yell at his or her family.

This is the great benefit of Aroma Reset - it allows us to remain in the flow of life by helping us to resolve current stressors without getting stuck in the feelings of hurt, frustration, anger, sadness or other emotions that may arise in the normal course of everyday life. By identifying and dealing with the situations that are causing us stress quickly and directly, we are more effective in solving our problems and moving in the direction of greater fulfillment.

In our Practitioner Certification Class, one of the first exercises I have the students do is a week of Aroma Resets - that is, I have them commit to doing an Aroma Reset every day consistently for a week, and then to notice the results.

Here are some of the comments the students have made after this exercise - these come directly from the feedback forms they fill out during class:

Reflection on doing Aroma Reset for a week
I noticed that doing a reset helps me get through my day without it being ruined by one unpleasant moment. I also usually have a hard time crying to release emotion/stress, that comes easily during a reset and passes quickly too. I feel lighter.

Reflection on doing Aroma Reset for a week
I love doing Aroma Reset each day. It really made it more possible to do all the things I need to do and not get stuck or overwhelmed. I feel much freer.

Reflection on doing Aroma Reset for a week
Feeling more excited, calm and confident with my life.

Reflection on doing Aroma Reset for a week
The reset has helped me personally with more focus and less wandering of my mind when I know I have important tasks to complete.

The 7 Day Aroma Reset Challenge

I invite you to experience this for yourself by committing to a "7 Day Aroma Reset Challenge." To do this, just choose a time (usually in the morning) to do your reset. Just think about your day, and let your mind review all of the things "on your plate." These could be upcoming commitments, such as a business meeting or family event, or they could be ongoing stressors, such as a project you have been working on for a while. They could also be recent events that you have found to be stressful or upsetting.

Once you have reviewed them, just choose one to do a reset on. Usually the most stressful thing on your mind will just pop into your consciousness when you start the process, so use that. You can do this while drinking your morning tea or coffee, meditating, sitting on the couch, or even in the shower (once you have memorized the steps)!

After your morning reset, you will likely feel energized and excited to start your day. Also, if you find yourself stressed or out of balance at any point during the day, just do another reset.

If you would like to experience the "7 Day Aroma Reset" with additional guidance, you are welcome to access our online program where I walk people through 7 days of Aroma Resets, complete with a facebook group, student support, and additional charts and resources. I hold these 7 day sessions live several times a year, and they can also be accessed through the recorded versions on demand.

To find out more, go to: www.aromafreedom.com/reset

Much of the power of the Aroma Reset comes from the increasingly accurate ability you will be developing of **naming feelings.** In fact, the ability to accurately describe and name your current emotional state has been correlated with greater emotional and mental health in general. This concept is called **"emotion differentiation,"** and it has been gaining increasing attention from scientists and researchers due to its importance in helping people with everything from managing depression to decreasing the likelihood of relapse of alcohol abuse. When we name an emotion, this begins to take away its power over us, primarily because emotions act like messengers in our bodies, urgently trying to give us messages about what situations mean to us. When we "receive the message," then the messenger is no longer needed, and we can focus on how we would like to respond to the message.

For instance, when you think about a specific situation and identify that you feel "overwhelmed," that is the first step towards deciding on a strategy to conquer it. Of course, when you do this using the full bodied approach contained within Aroma Freedom, you not only identify the feeling, but you also quickly shift it using the power of scent, and then have access to new guidance and wisdom about how to respond to the situation.

Several of the other variants of AFT - the "quick" techniques - build on the Aroma Reset and expand it into the future and the past. Keep reading to learn more!

Key Chapter Takeaways

The Aroma Reset Technique is a simple, 1-minute process for clearing the stress out of a current situation. It is based on the understanding that the same four aspects of a memory (image, feeling, body and thought) can be applied to the "image" of a current situation.

By doing an Aroma Reset on a situation, you can feel more relaxed and at-ease about it, and you may also receive guidance about how to proceed in that situation.

Even when you are feeling significant levels of overwhelm, frustration, confusion, or any other emotion, the Aroma Reset will quickly help you to focus on what is important, from a place of balance and calm.

Just do 1-2 rounds of Aroma Reset and then get on with your day.

Or, you may realize that a deeper technique is called for, such as AFT or TMRT.

Chapter 12

————— ⚜ —————

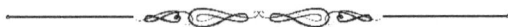

The Aroma Boost Technique: Antidote to Procrastination

"If anyone, then, knows the good they ought to do and doesn't do it, it is sin for them."

– The Bible, James 4:17

If you have tried the Aroma Reset introduced in the previous chapter, you probably have experienced how quickly and easily it transforms even quite distressing feelings such as overwhelm, frustration, or confusion into feelings of peace, calm, and even excitement about facing the formerly uncomfortable situations you encounter.

The Aroma Boost Technique builds on this experience and offers a specific way to channel the newly freed positive emotional energy into focused, inspired action to help you move forward in any area of your life in which you have been feeling stuck or stalled out.

Here are the steps:

The Aroma Boost Technique

	Step 1: Identify the Situation Think of a current situation that feels overwhelming, frustrating or confusing. Once you can clearly picture it, go to the next step.
	Step 2: Name the Feeling Find one word that describes how you feel when you picture the situation. Examples: sad, hopeless, lonely, fearful, etc.
	Step 3: Locate this feeling in your body Examples: Head, heart, belly, or anywhere else, or bodily posture such as feeling slumped over or teeth clenched. Once you have found it, go to the next step.
	Step 4: Identify the Negative Thought What is the negative thought connected to the feeling? Examples: "I don't have enough time" "I don't have enough money" "I am not smart enough"

	Step 5: Smell Essential Oils Place one drop each of Young Living Lavender, Frankincense, and Stress Away into your palms and rub together. Inhale deeply while focusing on the situation. Notice what happens to the picture of the situation, and to how you feel in your body and mind.
	Step 6: Decide what is next Now that something has shifted, you can either: A) Move on to the affirmation stage (step 7) B) Go back and clear another negative feeling (step 1) C) Take the time to do a full Aroma Freedom Session
	Step 7: Identify the next Action Step For the situation that had been previously overwhelming but is now feeling manageable, what is the next step needed in this situation?
	Step 8: Picture yourself doing the step and name the positive feeling you will have when it is done Examples: •Happy •Satisfied •Joyous •Grateful •…etc

	Step 9: Where do you feel this positive feeling in your body? Find where you feel this positive feeling – it could be in your: •Head •Heart •Smile •Belly •…or anywhere else!
	Step 10: Create an affirmation that integrates all of these elements: I feel _____ in my _____ as I _____. Examples: "I feel joy in my heart as I complete chapter 1 of my book today", or "I feel satisfaction in my smile as I call prospects I met at the expo yesterday"
	Step 11: Find a power pose that expresses the energy of this statement. Examples include "Victory," "Wonder Woman" or "Heart Centering" poses
	Step 12: Say your affirmation while smelling an essential oil and standing in your power pose Recommended Oils:•Transformation •Believe •Citrus Fresh •Lemon, or any Young Living Oil that you love.

Tips: Repeat the affirmation in the power pose 1 hour after the session to make sure you are still on track.

As with The Aroma Reset, I have all of my certification students do a week of Aroma Boosts on themselves and report on what they notice. Here is a small sampling of what they say:

Reflection on doing Aroma Boost for a week
I love doing Aroma Boost! They help get me out of a funk quickly and I feel energized to move productively through the rest of my day. Such a great tool!

Reflection on doing Aroma Boost for a week
Can I just say WOW!! It was amazing to have a tool to help me quickly resolve any frustrations that came up through the week. & Also to be able to serve others this way. I'm absolutely loving doing these sessions.

Reflection on doing Aroma Boost for a week
life is flowing smoothly and I'm able to be non-reactive more

Reflection on doing Aroma Boost for a week
It feels good to clear out old emotions and memories. Life isn't as tearful as its been lately. There is a feeling of being grounded.

After I started having students do a week of Aroma Boosts, I noticed that many of them reported suddenly being able to clean their offices, or check off their to-do lists, or just become more effective overall. I realized that the Aroma Boost is the perfect antidote to procrastination, because it helps people go from dreading or avoiding tasks, to eagerly embracing them. Let's dive a little deeper into the dynamics of procrastination to see why it works so well.

The Science of Procrastination and how Aroma Boost can help

In this section, I will review some of the science of procrastination, and then show how Aroma Boost is uniquely effective at resolving this very troubling and prevalent problem. In this way, you will see how something as simple as smelling the right oil, at the right time, with the right intention, can break you out of the prison of procrastination and into purposeful action.

For starters, we can define procrastination as **"the intentional or unintentional delay or avoidance of actions that you know will be beneficial to you."**

We have all experienced procrastination at some point in our lives. Recent research has identified that up to 80% of college students acknowledge that procrastination plays a significant role in their academic challenges. Furthermore, up to 20% of the general population has been identified as having problems with chronic procrastination.

Procrastination is often the BIGGEST problem standing in the gap between where you are and where you want to be. When you have a vision of how you want your life to go, goals you want to achieve, and projects you want to accomplish, it is necessary to **take action** to bring those dreams into reality. Failure to take inspired action is the formula for nothing changing in your life.

Researchers over the last 30 years have narrowed down most

257

problems of procrastination to two basic issues.

1. Task Aversiveness

2. Failure to consider future self-needs.

Let's take each in turn.

Task Aversiveness

It may seem obvious, but the main reason people procrastinate is because they imagine that the task they need to do will be unpleasant in some way. Psychologists call this "aversiveness," which can be defined as any stimulus that tends to cause someone to avoid something. In a laboratory example, imagine a lab rat that is given a small electric shock whenever he wanders over the left side of the cage, but no shock when he is in the middle or on the right. It won't take long before the rat will begin avoiding the left side of the cage - that location has become **aversive**.

The same is true for many things we encounter in life. Some experiences are pleasant, and some are unpleasant. We learn from our experiences, and, over time, develop an "inner map" of where to find the "goodies" of life - the pleasurable and enjoyable places, activities, and people whom we seek out. We also develop an "inner map" of what to avoid - situations that are painful (such as a bad trip to the dentist), frustrating (such as performing a new skill for which we are not adequately prepared), or lonely and sad (such as being alone on a friday night).

When we procrastinate, it is often because when we think about the task in question, we get an unpleasant feeling and so we avoid the task in order to avoid the unpleasant feeling. This has been referred to in the psychological literature as "short-term mood repair" - meaning, we do something to make ourselves feel better in the face of an unpleasant task (such as avoiding it or putting it off), rather than facing the task head-on.

Traditional wisdom has exhorted us to face problems "head-on" and "get things done" rather than avoiding and not doing them. In fact, here are several bible verses that point us in this direction:

"Whoever watches the wind will not plant; whoever looks at the clouds will not reap." **Ecclesiastes 11:4**

Interpretation: Take care not to just dream and think about things - this will not lead to concrete action and results. Rather, make sure to "plant" - (take action) in order to "reap" - experience results.

"No discipline seems pleasant at the time, but painful. Later on, however, it produces a harvest of righteousness and peace for those who have been trained by it." **Hebrews 12:11**

Interpretation: Doing the things we need to do in life is often not pleasant at the moment. However, the results that spring from these actions will be worth it later on.

"Lazy hands make for poverty, but diligent hands bring wealth." **Proverbs 10:4**

Interpretation: None needed.

The concept that there are many necessary actions that are unpleasant is fairly obvious. What is less obvious, however, is why these actions are judged to be so unpleasant. Why is it that a 5 year old child can gleefully "sweep the kitchen" with his or her mother, whereas the same person, as a 35 year old homeowner, finds every excuse to avoid housework? Or a teenager who spends hours fixing up a car but won't spend any time doing his or her homework?

There are many facets to this question, including a persons' overall preferences, skills, interests, areas of expertise, etc. The important point to consider at first, though, is that **every task that is "considered" to be unpleasant is first unpleasant in one's own mind.** It has frequently been noted that tasks are rarely as unpleasant as we imagine them to be beforehand.

When you imagine a task, you are projecting a level of pleasantness or unpleasantness to the task based on many factors, but primarily based on your **current mood** and your **past experiences**.

When you are in a bad mood, or struggling with depression, none of your favorite activities or tasks feel exciting. Have any of the activities themselves changed? Of course not. Your attitude has changed, and this affects whether you are able to imagine enjoying them or not.

Additionally, if you have done similar tasks in the past and have found them to be dull, boring, painful, humiliating, or negative in any way, that memory will feed into your assessment of the task at hand. You will project past failures into current projects, and (understandably) want to avoid them.

Your motivation to do a task depends on your current emotional state, whether you imagine the task itself to be pleasurable or painful **(aversiveness)**, and any perceived positive or negative outcome that will come from doing or **not** doing the task (see next section on embracing our future self).

You will remember that the miracle of memory reconsolidation using essential oils (TMRT and AFT) allows us to transform the feelings connected to unpleasant memories such that they no longer feel unpleasant.

Additionally, in the previous chapter we discovered that we could apply the same principles that we used with memories, and apply them to current situations (as in the Aroma Reset) such that current situations no longer carry a negative emotional charge as well.

What this means is that we now have a tool to reduce or eliminate the aversiveness of nearly any task. By reducing the aversiveness, we automatically increase our motivation to accomplish the task. Sometimes this involves improving our mood when considering the task so that it no longer seems so daunting, and sometimes it involves clearing out the memories that are connected to the proposed task so that they don't pollute our consideration of the task.

For example, I was recently working with one of the students in the Certification Class. Each week, the students are required to do a certain number of Aroma Freedom sessions on themselves as well as sessions on others. This is so that they become proficient in clearing out their own emotional baggage and integrating the Aroma Freedom tools into their daily lives.

One student, I will call her "Mary," was acknowledging that she had been able to deliver dozens of sessions to others, both individually and in groups, but had not yet been able to do any sessions on herself. She was embarrassed by this fact, as she clearly understood the steps of Aroma Freedom and was competent in delivering sessions. I decided to intervene and work with her in class, and the conversation went something like this:

Dr. Perkus: "I would like you to imagine doing an Aroma Freedom session on yourself." (This is Step 1 for Aroma Boost - picturing the task that is being avoided).

Mary: "OK, I got it."

Dr. Perkus: "What is the feeling that comes up when you picture this?" (Step 2)

Mary: "When I picture it, I feel sad and lonely"

Dr. Perkus: "Where do you feel these feelings in your body?" (Step 3)

Mary: "In my heart."

Dr. Perkus: "What is the negative thought that goes with those feelings?" (Step 4)

Mary: "I am all by myself, nobody cares."

Dr. Perkus: "OK, breathe your essential oils into this picture of doing a session on yourself and see what happens." (Step 5)

As Mary breathed into the imagined scenario, she began to tear up and cry. I allowed this to occur, encouraging her to just keep breathing the oils into the picture and noticing what happens. After a minute or two, the crying subsided, and she described what happened.

Mary: "It always goes back to the first memory of myself - when I was young and I was all by myself, nobody is home, I have been waiting and nobody's there. I have tears coming up from my heart."

Dr. Perkus: "OK, let's go into that a little bit. What is the feeling you get when you think about that memory?" (Doing another round of Reset/Boost, this time on the specific memory that came up).

Mary: "The feeling that comes up is 'I'm not lovable, I am not loved.'"

Dr. Perkus: "OK, those are the thoughts, what are the feelings?"

Mary: "I feel sad."

Dr. Perkus: "Where do you feel that sadness?"

Mary: "In my heart, in my chest."

Dr. Perkus: "OK, grab some 'Inner Child' oil blend, and breathe into that memory some more. You are doing great."

Mary breathes into the memory for a minute, then speaks.

Mary: "I am still at that memory. I hear a voice like it is my adult self speaking to my baby self, saying 'It's ok, I love you....they don't mean to not love you, it is just that they don't notice that you are waiting.' I feel less tense, not so tight."

Dr. Perkus: "OK, just keep breathing into the memory until it has gone as far as it is going to."

Mary: "Many of my AFT sessions go back to this memory."

Dr. Perkus: "How do you feel now when you picture the memory?"

Mary: (Considers this for a few moments, then starts to smile and her mood brightens) "I don't need to live there anymore. I can fly out. I don't need to stay there waiting!"

Dr. Perkus: "Now when you think about doing an Aroma Freedom session on yourself, how do you feel?"

Mary: "I think I can do it, but the feeling of going through it all by myself...I am scared of what will come out and nobody will be there to know what is going on with me. Deep down I feel I am desperate for some companionship, some working-togetherness. I know I am capable of doing it, but I am just reluctant to do it because I would like to do it with someone who will accompany me."

Dr. Perkus: "So you are more aware of the issues now. The feeling you just mentioned was fear, which is a little different than being sad and alone, so that tells me it is worth doing another round...where do you feel that fear in your body?" (Going to another round of Aroma Boost).

Mary: "Upper chest/throat. It is a horrifying and terrifying feeling."

Dr. Perkus: "And what is the negative thought that goes with that feeling?"

Mary: "It doesn't work...there is no point in doing it."

Dr. Perkus: "OK, take the 'trauma life' oil blend and breathe into that image of doing a session by yourself...what do you notice?"

Mary: (After a moment) "I notice me saying to myself...'I am my best company. I don't need anyone there. I can be powerful and use that power."

Dr. Perkus: "Great! So, how do you feel now about doing a session on yourself?"

Mary: "I will do it!" (Excited, empowered, smiling).

* * * * *

We will return to this session later in the chapter to see how the session ends.

For now, I would like to highlight the fact that Mary was able to go from thinking about a task that was aversive to her (doing an AFT session on herself) to being able to consider doing it without any feeling of aversion.

Importantly, we made no assumptions about what was going to be the aversive part of the task. As the work with her unfolded, it became evident that the thought of doing a session on herself triggered an early memory of being left all alone with no one to care for her. We needed to clear this memory in order for her to come back into the present moment and be able to consider the task without that emotional baggage attached to it.

When a task is aversive, there are an infinite number of reasons why it may be aversive. We just follow the Aroma Freedom process and let those reasons emerge and then get cleared away.

So the first part of the Aroma Boost is actually the same as the Aroma Reset you just learned in the last chapter, with the focus being specifically on a task that you are procrastinating on - one that is aversive for some reason and you have been avoiding or delaying.

Once you have performed the first part of Aroma Boost (Steps 1-6), you are ready to move to the second part (Steps 7-12).

Essentially, the formula for Aroma Boost is:

[Aroma Reset]

+

[Action Activator Affirmation]

After clearing out the aversiveness of the task with the Aroma Reset, you now will be installing an affirmation that specifically helps you to identify the positive feeling you will experience when you have done the action step.

Before we discuss the second half of Aroma Boost, though, let's return to the second aspect that has been identified as a critical piece in the puzzle of procrastination.

Failure to consider future-self needs

Procrastination is intimately connected with time. In every case of procrastination, there is an aspect of "putting it off into the future."

"I'll do it tomorrow."

"I will do it when I have time."

"The project isn't due for another two weeks."

"I'll do it when I get around to it."

In fact, according to Google, the word "procrastinate" is derived as follows:

late 16th century: from Latin *procrastinat-* 'deferred till the morning', from the verb *procrastinare*, from *pro-* 'forward' + *crastinus* 'belonging to tomorrow' (from *cras* 'tomorrow').

There is an implicit belief in every act of procrastination that you will be more in the mood to do the task tomorrow than you are today. Of course, this is rarely true. In fact, humans are notoriously bad at what psychologists call "affective forecasting." You may tend to imagine your happiness level in the future to be greater than it actually will be. People who hope they will win the lottery believe they will be happier after such a win, yet repeated studies show this not to be the case. On the other hand, people also may believe that they will be more miserable in the future than they are now - for instance during a painful relationship breakup, you may feel that you will never be happy again. Yet, after the dust settles, you generally return to whatever baseline of happiness you usually have.

The point is, thinking that you will "magically" be more in the mood to do an aversive task tomorrow is unlikely. It is usually the case that tasks that are put off are only accomplished eventually because of the **time pressure** to do them. As the deadline looms ever-closer, the pressure to act increases, such that eventually this pressure overpowers our resistance to the aversiveness of the task. Such is the power of deadlines - they "force our hand" so to speak and make us perform whether we like it or not. In fact, Tony Robbins once said "Goals are just dreams with a deadline."

Psychologists have called our tendency to be less motivated by distant goals than immediate goals "time discounting." The further away a goal is, the less impact it generally has on our level of motivation.

Researcher Piers Steel, in his classic review article entitled "The Nature of Procrastination: A Meta-Analytic and Theoretical Review of Quintessential Self-Regulatory Failure," described his "Temporal Motivation Theory" (TMT) as an integrative way to take both the aspects of enjoyment of a task as well as the time dimension into account to show how they both help to predict a person's tendency to procrastinate.

In this article, he gives the example of a fictional student "Thomas Delay." Thomas has been assigned a paper that is due on December 16. Seeing as it is only the beginning of September, the assignment seems so far away that it does not carry much weight in his consideration of whether to start writing versus going out and socializing with his friends. As October rolls around, the due date is still so far away that socializing easily trumps writing in his decision process. November brings more of the same - there is a gnawing feeling that he should begin, but still does not seem as relevant as the local party. Finally there comes a point in early December where the lines converge, and then, all of a sudden, working on the paper becomes more motivating than going to the next party. From that point forward, he works feverishly to finish the paper and hand it in just under the wire.

From the perspective of TMT, the desire to accomplish a task is roughly equivalent to:

[Enjoyment/value of the task]

divided by

[Length of time in the future that the consequences of doing the task will be experienced]

If the reward for doing a task (or the punishment for not doing it) is far off in time, it is difficult to feel motivation to accomplish it - just as Thomas Delay's paper would not lead to a reward or punishment until several months after it was assigned.

According to this formula, the only way to increase motivation to do a task will either be to

1. **Increase** the enjoyment or the value of the task.

or

2. **Collapse the expected time delay** of the consequences of doing the task to as close to zero as possible.

As previously mentioned, we know we can increase the enjoyment or value of the task by using the first part of the Aroma Boost and decreasing the **aversiveness** of the task using essential oils.

In order to collapse the expected time delay, we will be doing two things in the second half of the Aroma Boost:

1. Break the task into smaller sub-tasks that are due more quickly. We do this in Aroma Boost by identifying the **next step needed** to move toward the goal. This is a well tested strategy to accomplish big goals by breaking them into steps. Since each step is due sooner than the entire goal, the motivation to accomplish it will be higher.

2. Make the positive consequences of taking action as tangible and as immediate as possible (effectively

collapsing the time delay down to zero). You do this in Aroma Boost by identifying the positive feeling you will get when the task is accomplished and then imagining it, feeling it as viscerally as possible in your body, stating this out loud in a power pose while smelling oil. By mentally transporting yourself to the end point in your imagination, you have eliminated the time delay.

Just as we are manipulating aversiveness in our imagination with part one of the Aroma Boost, we are also manipulating time delay in our imagination in part two of the Aroma Boost.

As you can see on the instruction sheet, the second half of the Aroma Boost starts by identifying and picturing the next step needed in moving towards accomplishing the goal. Then, as you picture it, you identify the positive feeling you will get by doing it. Most people will feel this as something like pride, relief, happiness, joy, etc. You anchor this even more deeply by finding where you hold that positive feeling in your body.

Now you will combine all of these aspects into a specially formulated affirmation: "I feel _____ in my _____ as I _____"

For instance, "I feel joy in my heart as I finish the next chapter of my book," or "I feel relief in my spine as I finally tell my husband the secret I have been holding."

Let's return to the case of Mary, who was having trouble doing sessions on herself. We had cleared some memories that had been holding her back, and now wanted to make sure that she carried the change out into the world.

In the session, I suggested some possible affirmations or questions that she could use to help anchor that change. She thought about it for a minute, then composed the following Aroma Boost affirmation:

Mary: "I feel excited and powerful in my heart when I do AFT on myself."

In this way, she was able to connect the future expectation of feeling powerful with the task of doing AFT on herself. This made her excited and motivated to do it. She became visibly more animated and happy as she repeated this phrase over and over, smelling her Transformation oil blend.

The **action activator affirmation** that we do in the Aroma Boost brings completion to any clearing, and generates positive momentum towards our goals and projects.

In case you are wondering whether simply imagining doing a task has any effect on your emotions, consider this: Researchers at the National Institutes of Health (NIH) published a study in 2007 showing that remembering past episodic memories uses many of the same brain pathways as imagining future events.[7] In particular, the more you "elaborate" the imagined future event, the more likely your brain will be to treat it like a "real"

---

[7] Addis, Wong, and Schacter (2007): "Remembering the past and imagining the future: common and distinct neural substrates during event construction and elaboration." *Neuropsychologia*, 2007 April 8 45(7): 1363-1377

memory and respond emotionally to it.

The results of doing the Aroma Boost are remarkable, both in terms of how quickly it resets your motivation, and how excited you are to tackle tasks that had formerly felt onerous.

Give it a try and let us know what your results are!

Other aspects of Procrastination

Procrastination has been associated with a number of other psychological issues. Most of these, in the end, boil down to the various reasons why a task is seen as "aversive" in the first place, and for that reason, they can be fairly easily resolved using the different Aroma Freedom techniques.

For instance:

Perfectionism

Sometimes, people can't complete a task because they have such high standards for the task, it can never be seen as done well enough to move on to something else. For instance, when I was writing my first book in 2016, I was painfully aware that in order for me to reach my deadline, I would need to accept the fact that I would be publishing and selling a book with my name on it that was flawed in some way. This was not easy, but I came to the conclusion that it was better to release a good book that was imperfect than to release no book at all.

Upon reflection it is easy to see that I made the right choice - the thousands of people who have been helped by The Aroma

Freedom Technique would have never been reached if I held back until the book was "perfect" (which nothing can be).

If you find yourself struggling with doing or completing a project because of this issue, I suggest you do an AFT session on this issue. You can set your goal to be something like "I complete _____ task with ease and grace." If your negative voice that comes up says something about it not being perfect, just connect with the feeling that this statement triggers within you. It might be a feeling of shame, or pressure, or frustration. Whatever it is, just keep following the AFT process back to the bodily sensation and the memory that gets triggered. When you reconsolidate the memory by breathing essential oils into it, you will either get some specific guidance about the upcoming task, or your feeling state will soften into something more like peace, acceptance, or relaxation as you allow yourself to just do your best in the time allowed, and then move on.

Fear of Missing Out (FOMO)

If all of your friends are going to a party and you need to stay behind to write a paper, your FOMO will likely kick in. Just do an Aroma Boost by focusing on the paper you need to write and notice the feelings. They could be related to loneliness, sadness (of missing out on something good), resentment ("why do I have to be the only one left behind?"), boredom (Math is so boooooorrrrring!!), etc.

Allow yourself to feel these feelings. Find them in your body. Connect with these thoughts. Then breathe the essential oils into the picture of writing the paper. See what happens. It will probably break one of two ways. You might relax into the thought of writing the paper. Then the boost affirmation can help you to become excited about doing it. Or, the feeling may melt and along with it, you relax into a realization that you actually can go to the party - that trying to stay home and write the paper are not actually what your system needs right now.

In either case, you are no longer in conflict. You either enjoy the paper or enjoy the party!

Low Self Confidence

One of the reasons people don't do things is because they don't feel confident they can be successful at them. This may not be apparent at first, especially to an outsider. It is common for us to label people as "lazy" when we see them dawdling, not doing their chores, not taking actions they should take. Why is my son not doing his math homework? It could be because he would "rather" play video games (who wouldn't?), but it could also be because he does not feel confident that he can understand the material. Of course, like most children, he "acts out" his feelings rather than expressing them directly.

In this case, just naming the feeling is half the battle.

Father: "How do you feel when you think about doing your math homework?"

Son: "I don't know." (Most common answer from kids).

Father: "Let's see…angry, hopeless, confused, overwhelmed, frustrated…"

Son: "Yeah, frustrated."

Father: "Where do you feel that in your body?"

Son: "My jaw is tight."

Father: "What is the negative thought that goes with that frustration?"

Son: "My teacher goes too fast through the lessons."

Father: "OK, smell this oil and picture yourself doing the homework. See what you notice."

Son: (After just a few seconds...kids process really fast) "My jaw relaxed and I realized I need to speak up and tell the teacher to slow down when I don't understand."

Father: "Great! Can you picture yourself talking to your teacher about that? How will that feel?"

Son: "A little nervous but also excited."

Father: "Where do you feel that in your body?"

Son: "In my stomach."

Father: "What is the thought that goes with the nervous/excited feeling?"

Son: "I hope he listens to me."

Father: "OK. Breathe these essential oils into the picture of you talking to the teacher."

Son: (After a few seconds) "The picture changed and I saw us talking about math and then about other stuff too, and it was really relaxing and cool." (son smiles)

Father continues to lead his son through the affirmation part of the Aroma Boost, and they end up with the following affirmation:

"I feel excited in my heart as I speak to my teacher about the pace of the class."

You can see how a person's resistance to a task is frequently related to a worry or concern that is not obvious to someone on the outside.

You can also see that for almost any reason that is stopping you from doing a task, you can just follow the Aroma Freedom process to determine the underlying causes (often a negative thought process or memory of a previous incident), and then you use the essential oils to quickly shift either the memory or the perception of the task itself. We don't need to develop elaborate theories as to why you aren't following through on your actions or your goals - just follow the steps and let the technique take care of the rest!

If you would like to go deeper into using Aroma Freedom and Aroma Boost for Procrastination, go to
www.aromafreedom.com/procrastination
to access Dr. Perkus' masterclass in which he goes deeper into the science of why and how Aroma Freedom tackles

procrastination. In that class, you will also have the opportunity to experience a clearing related to any area in which you are procrastinating.

Key Chapter Takeaways

The Aroma Boost Technique is an elaboration of the Aroma Reset Technique. It involves one or two rounds of Aroma Reset, followed by a special affirmation that names the positive feeling you will have when you do the next action step needed in that situation.

Aroma Boost is an antidote to procrastination because it tackles the two main causes of procrastination:

1 - Task Aversiveness: You avoid tasks that you believe will be unpleasant in some way. Aroma Boost begins by identifying and clearing the negative feelings connected with thinking about the task. This places you in the mood to do the task and erases your reluctance to act.

2 - Time Discounting: You resist doing tasks whose consequences seem far away. Aroma Boost conquers this by connecting you with the positive feelings you will have when the next action step is completed. By doing the special Action Activator Affirmation, you are excited and ready to jump into action!

Other causes of procrastination, such as Perfectionism, Fear of Missing Out (FOMO), or Low Self Confidence, are also easily handled with the various Aroma Freedom Techniques.

Chapter 13

⸺⸺⸺ ❧❧❦❧❧ ⸺⸺⸺

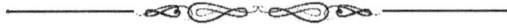

The Aroma Wisdom Technique: Antidote to Worry

"Wisdom cannot be imparted. Wisdom that a wise man attempts to impart always sounds like foolishness to someone else ... Knowledge can be communicated, but not wisdom. One can find it, live it, do wonders through it, but one cannot communicate and teach it."

— *Hermann Hesse, Siddhartha*

In April of 2020, near the beginning of the Covid-19 Pandemic, I found myself, like everyone else, trying to figure out what the heck was going on with our world. I had been watching Youtube videos, and listened to one in which the speaker was predicting that we would be falling into a dystopian future, kind of like the "Hunger Games," wherein everyone would be reduced to a paltry existence while the elites ruled over us with an iron fist.

The following day, I woke up depressed. This was notable for me, since I generally am a very optimistic and upbeat person, and have had lots of experience transforming negative emotions into positivity and growth.

I realized that my depressed mood was related to the images still floating in my head from the previous night, of mobs of hungry people swarming the countryside and fighting with each other, while the overlords look on for their entertainment.

I reasoned that these negative images of a possible future were not really much different from images that I knew could be successfully dismantled and dissolved from the past using The Memory Resolution Technique (TMRT) discussed earlier in this book.

So, always being my own guinea pig first, I tried an experiment. I did a session on myself but instead of the starting point being a disturbing memory (as in TMRT) or a disturbing current situation (as in Aroma Reset), I had the starting point be the upsetting imagined future that I had been thinking about.

As I imagined the upsetting future, I named the feeling that it evoked - depression. I found it in my body (heart). I identified the negative thought connected with the depressed feeling - that we are all going to be starving peasants ruled by tyrants. Then I just breathed the essential oils into the image of this future situation. After just a few moments, the image broke apart, and I came back to the present moment. I no longer felt depressed. My feeling shifted to curiosity. I realized that, while it is **possible** that this may be our future, that possibility does not need to define how I feel or live my life now. I regained my sense of creativity and the sense that I can choose how I want to live and spend my energy today, rather than being just weighed down by a future that may or may not ever occur.

I realized that a new technique had just been born. I called it the "Doomsday Technique," because that seemed to capture the starting point of the feeling of "Doom" that I had just liberated myself from. Over time, however, with the help of my students, I renamed it the "Aroma Wisdom" technique, because an inner guidance seems to always replace the image of the feared future that was previously there.

Here are the steps of The Aroma Wisdom Technique:

The Aroma Wisdom Technique

	Step 1: Identify the Feared Future Scenario or worry Think of a feared future worst-case scenario or worry, either personal or global. Once you can clearly picture it, go to the next step.
	Step 2: Name the Feeling Find one word that describes how you feel when you picture the scenario. Examples: sad, hopeless, lonely, fearful, etc.
	Step 3: Locate this feeling in your body Examples: Head, heart, belly, or anywhere else, or bodily posture such as feeling slumped over or teeth clenched. Once you have found it, go to the

	next step.
	Step 4: Identify the Negative Thought What is the negative thought connected to the feeling? Examples: "I don't have enough time" "I don't have enough money" "I am not smart enough"
	Step 5: Smell Essential Oils Place one drop each of Young Living Lavender, Frankincense, and Stress Away (or Trauma Life Oil by itself) into your palms and rub together. Inhale deeply while focusing on the situation. Notice what happens to the picture of the situation, and to how you feel in your body and mind.
	Step 6: Decide what is next If there is still an emotional charge when picturing the scenario, go back to step 1 and clear another feeling. If there is no more emotional charge, move to step 7.

	Step 7: Identify the next Action Step For the situation that had been previously worrisome but is now feeling manageable, what is the next step needed in this situation?
	Step 8: Picture yourself doing the step and name the positive feeling you will have when it is done Examples: •Happy •Satisfied •Joyous •Grateful •…etc
	Step 9: Where do you feel this positive feeling in your body? Find where you feel this positive feeling – it could be in your: •Head •Heart •Smile •Belly •…or anywhere else!
	Step 10: Create action or attitude affirmations, as desired: Action: I feel _____ in my _____ as I _____. Attitude: Create an "attitude affirmation" that expresses the wisdom and guidance you just received. Make a statement that integrates these affirmations, if desired.

	Step 11: Find a power pose that expresses the energy of this statement. Examples include "Victory," "Wonder Woman" or "Heart Centering" poses
	Step 12: Say your affirmation while smelling an essential oil and standing in your power pose Recommended Oils:•Transformation •Believe •Citrus Fresh •Lemon, or any Young Living Oil that you love.

Tips: Repeat the affirmation in the power pose 1 hour after the session to make sure you are still on track.

Keep doing the actions and affirmations until the problem is resolved.

Aroma Wisdom was originally created to deal with feelings of doom, hopelessness, or worry connected with the world - the images of armageddon related to nuclear war, climate disaster, pandemic, mass starvation, asteroids hitting the earth, and so on.

Early on, however, I realized that the technique was equally applicable to the more personal form of worry that we are all prone to in life - worry about ourselves, our children, family, friends, etc. When you worry, you are projecting a negative future into your imagination, and then responding emotionally to that picture. This is the case when you think of the "worst case scenario" for any upcoming situation. It could be worry that you will get into a car accident, worry that you will lose your job and become homeless, worry that your kids will get sick, worry that the roof will start leaking and you won't be able to afford a fix, and so on.

We tend to do this automatically, without knowing that we are creating such an image. Therefore, the first step to working with worry using Aroma Wisdom is to actually take the time to picture and consciously imagine what you are worried about. Ask yourself "What is the worst case scenario?" This is what you are emotionally responding to. Once you have the picture, you can simply follow the familiar steps to working with it - name the feeling, find it in your body, connect the negative thought related to the feeling, and then breathe essential oils (Trauma Life, Inner Child, or Memory Release Blend) into the imagined future scenario.

You will likely find the image quickly dissolving, and in its place, you may become aware of some inner guidance about the situation at hand. I find that the future imagined scenario tends to dissolve more quickly than, for instance, a traumatic memory that you might work with in TMRT. Although they are both images, the future image has been constructed entirely in your imagination, whereas the past image has been consolidated over years of inner rehearsal and is therefore a little more stable and takes a little longer to dislodge.

Here is an example with one of my students (we will call her

Molly) on using Aroma Wisdom on a personal worry.

Dr. Perkus: "Think of something you worry about."

Molly: "I am always worried that my 6 year old son will drown in our backyard swimming pool. I can't even enjoy being out there because I am so tense."

Dr. Perkus: "Picture the worst case scenario - what do you see happening?"

Molly: "I see him falling in the water and flailing his arms and crying out." (emotions begin to surface for Molly)

Dr. Perkus: "What is the one word feeling you get when you picture this?"

Molly: "Terror."

Dr. Perkus: "Where do you feel the terror in your body?"

Molly: "In my chest…it is hard to breathe."

Dr. Perkus: "What is the negative thought that connects with the feeling of terror?"

Molly: "I won't be able to save him."

Dr. Perkus: "Breathe the Trauma Life oil into that image of him flailing in the water."

Molly: (after a minute of breathing the oil) "The feeling of terror is gone. But now I just feel worried that it isn't safe."

Dr. Perkus: "OK, let's do another round on that. Where do you feel the worry in your body?"

Molly: "In my head."

Dr. Perkus: "What is the negative thought that connects with that worry?"

Molly: "The pool just isn't safe."

Dr. Perkus: "Breathe the Inner Child oil into that image of him in the pool and notice what happens."

Molly: (after just a few moments) "The image dissolved and the idea just popped into my head that I should sign him up for swimming lessons!" (smiles)

Dr. Perkus: "Great! So how do you feel now about the image of him drowning in the pool?"

Molly: "I can't even really see that image any more. Now I am just thinking of where I can get him swimming lessons and feeling excited to see him learn how to swim!"

We went on to create a plan for her to contact the YMCA and get him enrolled and she did an affirmation to anchor this action plan in place.

This example highlights several important features of Aroma Wisdom and how to process worry.

1. The initial image was something that has never happened, but which was still generating significant

distress whenever she thought about it.

2. Highlighting the "worst case scenario" brought the emotion to the surface, thus allowing her to process it effectively.

3. The first round of clearing brought the feeling intensity down and changed it slightly - she went from "terrified" to "worried." Whenever you do multiple rounds of clearing, always name the new feeling that is surfacing, as it may be different than the original feeling.

4. We switched oils for the second round. This is not always necessary, but sometimes it can be helpful to smell a new oil just to keep the processing moving.

5. After the emotional distress subsided in the second round, Molly spontaneously heard a voice of wisdom and got an inspired thought about how to proceed in this situation.

6. Once we were done, she could barely see the original upsetting image, and instead felt excited to follow through with her action plan that not only would reduce the chances that her son would drown, but would actually give him a new skill and would even be fun!

Where does the "voice of wisdom" come from in this technique? That is a mystery. We could call it the "Voice of Reason," the "Higher Self," the "Holy Spirit," or just "Common Sense." We may never know the answer to that question.

To be clear, the "voice of wisdom" emerges in just about every Aroma Freedom session, no matter which particular technique you are using. In the 12-step AFT process, wisdom comes in the form of your new attitude towards your goal. In Aroma Boost, it is an inspired action step that you will do to move forward. In TMRT, it can be a gentle voice whispering to you that you are "OK" instead of being trapped in a traumatic situation from your memory. In all of these cases, the **wisdom emerges spontaneously once the emotional charge has been released.** Importantly, we as practitioners never tell the client what they "should" think about a situation. Rather, we allow the answer to emerge from within. If we try to give "advice" about a situation, it will always be coming from outside and might not be the right answer for the client, even though it makes logical sense.

The Aroma Wisdom Technique is the method of choice whenever you, or your clients, are having feelings of worry, doom, or dread about the future - whether it is the future of our world, or the future for themselves or their loved ones. It can be used as a stand-alone technique, in these cases. It also can be used at any point during a session when you (or your client) begin worrying about a future outcome. Just picture the worrisome situation, and follow the rest of the steps in the technique.

To watch a video demonstration of this technique, visit www.aromafreedom.com/wisdom

Key Chapter Takeaways

The Aroma Wisdom Technique was created in response to the uncertainty and worry that the pandemic was bringing in 2020.

A key insight was that the "image of the worrisome future" can be processed in the same way that the "past images" are processed in TMRT, or the "current images" are processed in Aroma Reset and Aroma Boost.

The steps for Aroma Wisdom are the same as that of the Aroma Boost - the only difference is starting from the imagined future rather than the current situation.

Aroma Wisdom can be used for personal worries (about your kids, yourself, finances, health, or anything else) as well as for global worries (what is happening in the world, where is our country heading, will there be a nuclear war, etc.)

When processing upsetting future imaginings using Aroma Wisdom, pay close attention to any words of wisdom, new perspectives, inner guidance, or anything else that may emerge spontaneously during the session. This will be your key to the right attitudes and actions for you to navigate the situation.

Chapter 14

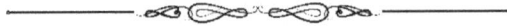

The Aroma Clear Technique and Hybrid Sessions

"Memories are the key not to the past, but to the future."

— *Corrie Ten Boom*

Before we discuss the final technique, let's review the previous five Aroma Freedom Techniques.

The first two techniques - Aroma Freedom Technique (AFT) and The Memory Resolution Technique (TMRT) - involved, in various ways, finding and clearing the emotional charge connected with **past memories.**

The next three techniques - Aroma Reset, Aroma Boost, Aroma Wisdom - involved clearing the emotional charge for **current or future situations**.

The Aroma Clear technique creates a bridge between the two realms of the **present and the past.**

As we have discussed throughout this book, many of your emotional reactions to current situations really originate in unresolved situations from the past. The Aroma Clear is especially helpful for the problem of "overreaction."

The Problem of Overreaction

Imagine the following scenario:

You are settling down to bed when your spouse asks you, in a calm voice, "Did you remember to take out the garbage?"

"NO!" you shout, suddenly agitated. "Why do I have to do everything around here???"

You get up and angrily put on your robe, trudge out to the curb with the garbage can, then come back inside to bed in a huff, and silently begin to read your book.

"Why are you in such a bad mood?" your spouse asks.

"You are always on me about something!" you respond.

"I wasn't criticizing you, I was just trying to remind you about the garbage," your spouse says.

…and so the fight begins.

What just happened?

Ideally, everyday life events should trigger emotional responses that are appropriate to the situation. When you are unfairly criticized, it is appropriate to feel angry. When you have to say goodbye to your loved ones after a holiday visit, it is normal to feel sad. When you hear a sound downstairs in the middle of the night, it is understandable that you would feel afraid, at least until you discover it is just the cat knocking over a vase and not an intruder.

However, we have all experienced reactions that are not so straightforward. We get flustered and panicked over a minor delay. We yell at our kids over a minor mistake. We feel devastated when our partner forgets something we told them.

Overreaction occurs when the emotional response to a situation is out of proportion to what the situation calls for.

How can essential oils possibly help with this? We will get to that in a moment.

The first thing to understand is where this excess emotional response is coming from. As you might imagine, your brain has been keeping a tally of the various slights, hurts, and injustices you have experienced throughout your life. When you assess a current situation, you are not just seeing what is happening in the present moment. You are seeing it through the filter of all the other experiences you have had. Importantly, you are connecting past memories of similar times through the lens of feeling, not necessarily context. This means that when your spouse corrects you, this activates not just all the other times that he or she has corrected you, but also all of the times that anyone has corrected you. Not only that, it will activate the memory patterns of times when you have been unfairly attacked, criticized, or mistreated.

When this happens, it can create an emotional response that is out of proportion to the current situation. You "snap."

Of course, at that moment, you are not aware of the past events, you are just focused on the current trigger and how "irritating" it is.

This tendency to be "triggered" by current situations can have unfortunate consequences. By overreacting to a current stressor and screaming about a situation that does not warrant it, this creates a domino effect whereby the other person will, correctly, feel that they do not deserve this intense response. They may, in turn, become triggered and raise their emotional intensity to your level or even higher.

We see this regularly in intimate relationships. A spiral of escalating emotional intensity quickly devolves into name calling, unfair attacks, dredging up the past, and even in some cases, physical violence. In fact, according to the Proceedings of the Mayo Clinic (1998), domestic partner violence is the leading cause of injury to women aged 15 - 44, and the second leading cause of injury to women overall. In my work as a therapist for many years, I have needed to teach couples how to "fight fairly" by communicating effectively, and to recognize and avoid the spiral of escalation.

Thus it is very important that we have a method to "unwind" this emotional buildup and to resolve the roots of what can otherwise become an intractable and potentially dangerous situation. Even if you are not in a situation that has become aggressive or violent due to unresolved emotional buildup, it is extremely useful to be able to clear away the excess reactivity in your life, so that you can find peace and happiness within the daily stressors of life.

Here are the steps of the Aroma Clear Technique:

The Aroma Clear Technique

	Step 1: Identify a situation that "triggers" you Think of a current situation that makes you reactive, upset, or triggered into intense emotion. Once you can clearly picture it, go to the next step.
	Step 2: Name the Feeling Find one word that describes how you feel when you picture the situation. Examples: sad, hopeless, lonely, fearful, etc.
	Step 3: Locate this feeling in your body Examples: Head, heart, belly, or anywhere else, or bodily posture such as feeling slumped over or teeth clenched. Once you have found it, go to the next step.

	Step 4: Identify the Negative Thought What is the negative thought connected to the feeling? Examples: "I don't have enough time" "I don't have enough money" "I am not smart enough"
	Step 5: Memory Drift back to an earlier time when you felt the same way. Notice the first memory or image that pops up, from recently or long ago. It could be a snapshot of a specific time, or a "movie" multiple times.
0-10	**Step 6: Rate the Emotional Charge** Rate how intense the feeling is when you picture that memory, from 0=No Emotional Charge, to 10=Most Intense Possible.
	Step 7: Smell Essential Oils Place one drop each of Young Living Lavender, Frankincense, and Stress Away into your palms and rub together. Inhale deeply while focusing on the memory. Notice what happens.

	Step 8: Repeat the process until no more charge If there is still an emotional charge when picturing the memory, rate the memory again (0-10) and then go back to steps 2, 3, 4 and identify the feeling, bodily sensation, and thought connected with the memory now (not the original situation). Smell essential oils again such as inner child or release oil to process the memory. Once there is no more emotional charge, move to step 9.
	Step 9: Picture yourself doing an action step and name the positive feeling you will have when it is done, also where you feel it in your body Examples: "Happy in my heart," "Confident in my smile"
	Step 10: Create action or attitude affirmations, as desired: Action: I feel _____ in my _____ as I _____. Attitude: Create an "attitude affirmation" that expresses the wisdom and guidance you just received. Make a statement that integrates these affirmations, if desired.

	Step 11: Find a power pose that expresses the energy of this statement. Examples include "Victory," "Wonder Woman" or "Heart Centering" poses
	Step 12: Say your affirmation while smelling an essential oil and standing in your power pose Recommended Oils:•Transformation •Believe •Citrus Fresh •Lemon, or any Young Living Oil that you love.

Tips: Repeat the affirmation in the power pose 1 hour after the session to make sure you are still on track.

Keep doing the actions and affirmations until the problem is resolved.

As you may have noticed, the Aroma Clear is really a combination of the Aroma Reset (starting with a current situation), and The Memory Resolution Technique (TMRT). Just like with the Aroma Reset, you are identifying a current situation, naming the feeling, finding it in your body, and identifying the negative thought. But instead of breathing the essential oils into the image of the current situation (as in the Aroma Reset), you will do one more critical step: You will drift back to an earlier time when you felt the same way. A picture will pop up either of a specific time, or a series of times, when you felt this way. You will breathe the essential oils into that memory, and watch what happens. Once back at the memory, you treat it just like you do in TMRT - rating the intensity, and then doing as many rounds of clearing as you need so that, when you think about the memory, there is no longer an emotional charge.

Once you have cleared the emotional charge, you return to the current situation and identify what the next appropriate action step is for the situation. In other words, once you are no longer being "triggered" by the situation, you are able to find the proper response without loading it up with all of your "baggage" from the past.

Example of Aroma Clear with a Couple:

I was working with a couple in therapy one time and the opportunity to use Aroma Clear came up. Let's call them Joe and Melissa. The conflict at hand was that when they were in the car, she would continually ask him to drive more slowly and carefully, and he would deny that there was anything wrong with his driving. She said he was reckless, and he said that she was being too controlling for no reason. As they discussed this issue in my office, their emotions were starting to escalate, with each partner attempting to make their point more and more forcefully. As I commented on this, they told me that they frequently had fights triggered by this issue and that it usually ended with name-calling, hurt feelings, frustration, and a period of uncomfortable silence.

I proposed that we do something a little different this time. I led them through an Aroma Clear exercise together. (This is one of the ways that the Aroma Freedom Techniques can be integrated into couples therapy. We discuss this in greater detail during the Practitioner Certification Training.)

The session went something like this:

Dr. Perkus: "I would like each of you to remember the last time you were in the car together and this issue came up. Don't say anything, just nod your head when you can picture it. Now, name the feeling you get when you picture that scene."

Joe: "Angry."

Melissa: "Scared."

Dr. Perkus: "Where do you feel that feeling in your body?"

Joe: "My teeth are clenched and I feel my fists squeezing a little."

Melissa: "I feel a tightness in the pit of my stomach."

Dr. Perkus: "And what is the negative thought you are having that connects to that feeling?"

Joe: "Why does she have to be so controlling?"

Melissa: "I feel out of control."

Dr. Perkus: "OK, now connect with that feeling - Anger for Joe, and Fear for Melissa - and drift back to an earlier time when you felt the same way. It could be a specific time like a snapshot, or a movie of the many times when you felt this way.

Joe: "I remember my mother always yelling at me to get up in time for the school bus. I felt tired, grumpy and angry that she was bothering me."

Melissa: "I remember my stepfather coming home drunk at night when I was a teenager, and feeling scared and desperate." (She begins to tear up).

Dr. Perkus: "OK, hold out your hands. Here is a drop of essential oil." (Placing a drop of Trauma Life oil blend in each of their hands.) "Breathe the oil into these memories and just notice what happens."

Joe and Melissa take a moment and breathe into the memories.

Dr. Perkus: "What did you notice?"

Joe: "As I breathed the oil into the memory, the whole scene softened and I realized that my mother was just trying to get me to school on time - the anger melted and I actually felt grateful that she was so insistent. I probably wouldn't have graduated if she had given up on me."

Melissa: "At first, when I was picturing that scene, I felt really scared. As I kept breathing the oil, it actually shifted to feeling angry that my stepfather was acting that way and that my mother would allow it."

Dr. Perkus: "OK, let's do another round. When you each picture that memory, what feeling do you have now?"

Joe: "I just feel peace and gratitude."

Melissa: "I am still feeling angry at my mom and step dad."

I led them through this second round, naming the bodily and mental aspects of the memories, and then smelling a different oil (Inner Child) into the memories. Then after a minute, asking what they each noticed.

Joe: "I relaxed even more, and I pictured myself as a teenager actually deciding to set an alarm and get myself up so that my mother didn't have to wake me up."

Melissa: "My anger intensified initially and I pictured myself yelling at my mom and step dad and telling them to get their act together. I wasn't afraid anymore. And then I pictured my step dad apologizing to us all and getting help for his drinking. I feel just kind of stunned and strangely calm now when I think about it."

Dr. Perkus: "Great! Now come back to the current situation. Picture yourselves in the car and he is driving faster than you want him to. What do you each feel now?"

Joe: "When I picture that now, I am able to hear her request to slow down without getting angry. I can see that she just wants to feel comfortable and not that she is trying to control me. I actually feel immature for having always taken it personally. I'm sorry, Melissa," he says, looking at her.

Melissa: "When I picture us in the car now, I feel stronger. I don't feel so out of control or scared. I can still see me asking him to slow down if it seems too fast for me, but I don't have the same desperate or panicked feeling. And I feel like he will listen to me better now because I know that I deserve to be treated with respect." She looks at him and the two of them hug.

In this session, each partner was able to connect with and transform the specific memories that were being triggered by the conversation. This brings up several points:

1. Although each partner was triggered and over-reacting, they were each triggered in their own unique way. For one it was anger, for the other it was fear.

2. The memories that were behind the over-reaction had nothing to do with the current situation in terms of context. Neither of the triggering memories were about riding in a car or going too fast. The memories were triggered by a similar **feeling**.

3. When the memories were activated in a full-bodied way and then essential oils were introduced, they spontaneously shifted into something new without input from the therapist and without the clients **trying** to feel any particular way.

4. When returning to the current situation, the clients did not need to try to feel anything differently about their partner. Again, there was a spontaneous new feeling and perception that arose. They were able to see the situation more clearly, without the filters from the past that had been affecting their previous perceptions and emotions.

5. By clearing out their reactivity, they were able to find a
   solution that empowered both of them.

We call this technique "Aroma Clear" because it enables "Clear Perception" in the current situation, unclouded by the hidden memories and reactions that had previously been running the show. As with all of the Aroma Freedom techniques, it uses the principle of Memory Reconsolidation to quickly shift the meaning and structure of the memory, allowing new perceptions, thoughts, and attitudes to come in.

It is appropriate to use Aroma Clear whenever it seems that your reactions or emotions feel out of control or inappropriate to the current situation.

This could be when you find yourself yelling (or crying) with your family at the drop of a hat. It could also be when you are feeling intense resentment about something that you have to do, or have a strong reaction to a new person or situation you are encountering. In short, it is wise to be suspicious that there may be triggering memories that have become activated in your daily life whenever you feel out of control. Using the Aroma Clear is a quick way to pull the problem out by the root so you can again have clear perception in the present moment.

A few more notes about Aroma Clear and Hybrid Sessions:

Sometimes, when doing an Aroma Reset or an Aroma Boost, you will spontaneously have a memory surface, without looking for it. When this happens, just follow the steps of the Aroma Clear and process the memory as I have outlined. Then, come back to the present and finish the Reset or the Boost. In fact, you can use Aroma Clear whenever a memory surfaces, OR whenever you suspect that there may be a memory underneath the issue that has been triggered.

This brings up a final point as we close out the discussion of the six Aroma Freedom Techniques:

Although the techniques are taught as separate processes, each with its ideal starting and ending point, the reality is that human beings are complex entities both psychologically and emotionally. There are times during any kind of Aroma Freedom session, when it will become apparent to the skilled practitioner that a new direction is called for. For instance, during a classic, 12-step AFT session, the memory that you are brought back to may not clear completely during the first round of processing. In such a case, I advise you to stay with that memory for several more rounds of processing (essentially going from "AFT" to "TMRT"), until the memory has lost its emotional charge. Then, simply return to the AFT process by going back to the goal statement and rating how possible it feels now. This is called a "AFT/TMRT" hybrid, and it happens fairly frequently in sessions. More training on hybrid sessions happens in the certification program. To discuss the program and see if it is right for you, book a call with me at www.aromafreedom.com/call

Key Chapter Takeaways

The Aroma Clear Technique is perfect for those situations in which you are "overreacting" to current stressors.

When you overreact, you are bringing the energy of unresolved past situations into your assessment of the current situation.

The Aroma Clear Technique starts with an Aroma Reset, but then has you drift back to an earlier time when you felt the same way.

After finding the triggering memory, just process it the way you would with TMRT.

Aroma Clear can be used at any point during a session, when it seems that there may be something from the past that is "driving" the current distress.

"Hybrid" sessions can occur during an Aroma Freedom session, when you spontaneously "stumble" into a past memory that does not quickly clear. In that case, you need to take some time to process the memory using TMRT, and then come back to the present.

Conclusion:
STARTING YOUR AROMA FREEDOM ADVENTURE

Chapter 15

Review and How to Move
Forward

"If you can't fly then run, if you can't run then walk, if you can't walk then crawl, but whatever you do you have to keep moving forward."

- *Martin Luther King Jr*

I hope you have enjoyed our time together as much as I have enjoyed writing this book for you!

The purpose of this chapter is to review what we have so far discussed in this book, and then look at how to best start using these techniques for your own personal transformation, whether by yourself or with the help of a practitioner, the Aroma Freedom Academy, or a mental health professional.

Book and Technique Overview

As I mentioned at the outset, Aroma Freedom was born out of my 20+ year quest to find simple and effective solutions for my clients that could also be easily taught to others so as to spread the healing power of what we were doing exponentially.

To review, here is what we covered in the book:

- Aroma Freedom helps people find freedom from painful memories, negative moods, powerlessness, paralysis, self doubt, and much more.

- Aroma Freedom provides a simple solution to the human tendency to get lost in complexity.

- Aroma is your most primitive and powerful sense, and connects directly with the limbic system of the brain, which is the seat of emotion and memory.

- Smelling Essential Oils is a well-researched method for quickly triggering strong mental and emotional responses and calming the limbic system.

- Memory (especially implicit memory) is one of the main drivers of your behavioral responses, and shapes how you respond to the challenges of life.

- Aroma Freedom brings the possibility of actually changing your memories - how they look, how they feel, and what they mean - and with that, changing your whole outlook on life. This is done using the natural brain process of "memory reconsolidation."

- Memory Reconsolidation in Aroma Freedom works by triggering a memory in all of its visceral fullness, and then introducing new "information" into the nervous system - namely, the powerful and irresistibly calming smell of an essential oil. This juxtaposition induces a re-writing of the neural pathways associated with the memory.

- There are six Aroma Freedom Techniques we covered in the book, each used with a slightly different intention. They are:

  o The Aroma Freedom Technique - To reach your goals

  o The Memory Resolution Technique - To clear negative memories

  o Aroma Reset - To stay in the flow of life

  o Aroma Boost - To end procrastination

  o Aroma Wisdom - To transform worry into wisdom

  o Aroma Clear - To end reactive emotions

- Finally, we discussed the importance of having the "spirit of freedom" and a "growth mindset" in order to make the whole system work for you.

Personal and Professional Application

As I mentioned in the beginning, I wrote this book for two audiences:

1. Individuals looking to overcome emotional, mental, health or life challenges, either through self-help or by

receiving services from a professional.

2. Professional therapists, coaches, and other practitioners who would like to add a powerful new tool to their toolbox of therapeutic methods for helping their clients.

Let's discuss each in turn:

For Individuals - Personal Use

This book is for people who are feeling held back by **inner obstacles** (doubt, worry, procrastination, anxiety, negative memories, etc.) or **outer obstacles** (difficult circumstances, unfulfilling relationships, financial problems, etc). In either of these cases, the Aroma Freedom Techniques offer a way forward by giving you the tools you need to dissolve and overcome such obstacles. All of the techniques can be used by yourself, on yourself. In many cases, this allows you to "pull yourself up by your own bootstraps," which is especially helpful when there is no one around to do it for you! It is also much more efficient to be able to help yourself out of a jam whenever you need to than to require someone else to help you.

Next Steps for Individual Use of Aroma Freedom:

1. If you don't yet have the essential oils and blends discussed in this book, contact us to get a sample kit sent to you at www.aromafreedom.com/oils - as soon as you have your oils, you can begin transforming yourself and others!

2. Try some of the techniques out on yourself using the

guides found in the earlier chapters of the book, or get full-color, laminated or downloadable guides here: www.aromafreedom.com/guides

3. Join our Aroma Freedom facebook group to connect with others learning these techniques, ask questions, and learn about upcoming trainings here: https://www.facebook.com/groups/1864614900439621

4. Follow along with guided sessions from Dr. Perkus and also participate in challenges and group interaction by joining the Aroma Freedom Training Vault here: www.aromafreedom.com/trainingvault

5. If you get great results using Aroma Freedom on yourself or others, and wish to become trained to do it professionally, you can learn more about Aroma Freedom Certification here by booking a call with me here: www.aromafreedom.com/call

When to seek out a Psychologist/Mental Health Professional:

Let me be clear that Aroma Freedom, by itself, is not a mental health therapy, and there are times when you need to seek professional help. You should seek help from a licensed mental health professional if any of the following apply to you:

1. You have been diagnosed with a mental disorder according to the DSM-5 (Diagnostic and Statistical Manual of Mental Disorders, Version 5). This could

include diagnoses such as major depression, post-traumatic stress disorder, or an anxiety disorder. It could also include personality disorders, schizophrenia, or autistic spectrum disorders. In such cases, it is important that you are under the care of a licensed professional who is trained to help you.

2. You are taking psychotropic medication, such as antidepressants, anti anxiety medications, etc.

3. You are having thoughts of harming yourself or others, or feel mentally or emotionally unstable.

4. Even if you have never been diagnosed with a mental disorder, but you find that you are having difficulty functioning in daily life, and that your symptoms are interfering with work, relationships, or taking care of yourself and your needs, you should seek the help of a licensed professional.

While you are receiving treatment from a mental health professional, Aroma Freedom Techniques can be used effectively as an adjunct to your counseling or therapy. If you are doing sessions on yourself, or having them done by a Certified Aroma Freedom Practitioner, just tell your therapist what you are doing, or sign a release and let them speak directly with the practitioner. Clients find that the combination of therapy and Aroma Freedom gives them the best of both worlds - someone to talk with to make sense of life and offer support (from the therapist), as well as fast relief from troubling memories and inner blocks to success (from the Aroma

Freedom Practitioner).

In fact, we encourage you to lend a copy of this book to your therapist - this will help him or her to understand what you are doing. Additionally, if your therapist wants to get trained in Aroma Freedom through our certification program, it could enhance his or her practice as well as your treatment!

For Professionals

Aroma Freedom was created as a result of decades of experience, training, and practical application of techniques in my clinical psychology practice. The Aroma Freedom Techniques are perfectly suited for use by psychologists and other mental health professionals. It is also a great addition to many types of coaching, education, and consulting. In short, if you have clients who get stuck emotionally in any of the ways we have been discussing, then Aroma Freedom can be a tool you can use to help them become free. Here is a quick visual of where Aroma Freedom might fit as a center point of integration between the realms of Psychology, Coaching, and Aromatherapy:

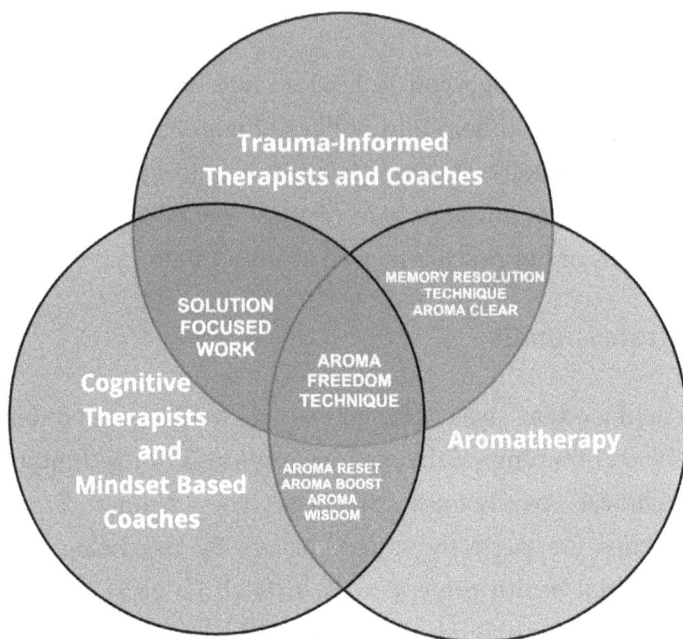

It can also be used adjunctively in a clinical practice such as medicine, chiropractic, massage therapy, acupuncture, etc. In such cases, Aroma Freedom can be delivered by the practitioner him or herself, or can be delivered by someone in your office specifically trained in the techniques. Since the role of unresolved emotion is well known as a driver of physical illness, it can be extremely beneficial to have someone versed in these techniques helping your clients or patients quickly resolve the underlying emotional pain that may be contributing to their illness.

Next Steps for Professional Use of Aroma Freedom:

Here is how to get started:

1. Use the techniques on yourself! See above list of resources for Individual Use to get started. I always tested techniques I was learning on myself first before using them on my clients.

2. Practice the techniques with family, friends, and colleagues. You will learn the power of the techniques first-hand and this will give you a level of competence before trying them with clients.

3. Join our facebook group created specifically for Mental Health Professionals here:
    https://www.facebook.com/groups/1926257894275047

4. Reach out to us to discuss becoming a Certified Practitioner. You must become certified if you would like to use the techniques professionally. You will experience tremendous personal growth in the program and become masterful at Aroma Freedom. It can become an additional revenue stream for you or someone in your practice. Schedule a call with us at www.aromafreedom.com/call and we will discuss training options. Don't worry, this is a no-pressure call. Since you have already read the book, you have a good idea of what we do and whether you want to be a part of it. If you are a good fit, we will be happy to welcome you to the group of 1000+ Practitioners who have been

trained since 2016. If not, that's ok too!

I wish you success and freedom on your journey, and hope someday to meet you in person or virtually and hear about your wins!

Sincerely,

Dr. Benjamin Perkus

Appendix

―――――――― ∞⟨⟩∞⟨⟩∞ ――――――――

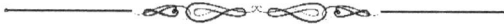

Essential Oils used in Aroma Freedom

"Essential Oils are little drops of God."

― **Dr. Wayne W. Dyer**

Author's note: Our Essential Oil Journey

As I had mentioned in the introduction, my wife, Elaine, and I began using essential oils many years ago, simply out of curiosity. We had always been interested in holistic and natural solutions, and in my Psychology practice I had already been integrating new modalities such as Resonance Repatterning, Emotional Freedom Technique (EFT), Neurofeedback, Eye Movement Desensitization and Reprocessing (EMDR), and more. Elaine was a natural networker and had brought many world-class healers and teachers to our home for classes and workshops on a variety of topics. Our first exposure to essential oils was at a class about Young Living Essential Oils (YLEO). Young Living was founded by Dr. Gary and Mary Young in 1993, and it works through the model of independent distributors enrolling and then teaching and supporting their customers, some of whom may choose to become distributors themselves.

Gary said that he chose this model of distribution (network marketing) because it has support and education baked right into the business model. If you purchase essential oils at a health food store it is very convenient, but once you get them home, there is no one to show you how to use them. However, when you get essential oils from a Young Living Independent Distributor, they will teach you how to use them, connect you with resources for learning, and help you connect with others for support as well.

Our experience when we became distributors was exactly like that. We had stepped into a world in which we had people who supported us in our learning, answered our questions, and taught us everything they knew (our upline). They came and taught in our house when we invited friends over. Eventually they encouraged us to teach our own classes. As interest grew and people continued to get wonderful results from the oils, we realized that we had developed a team of people who were traveling in the same direction as we were - towards empowerment, natural healing, and toxin-free living.

We also realized that we had, unwittingly, developed a business which gave us passive, residual income. We had not joined Young Living for the income - we just loved using the oils, and we also loved sharing them with others and having a community of like-minded people to learn and grow with. Once our monthly checks became large enough to get our attention, we began to take the business more seriously, but it always was, and still remains, about helping people and education first and foremost.

Throughout all of this, I still had my Clinical Psychology practice, which I loved. By day, I saw clients in my therapy office connected to the front of our house. On nights and weekends, my wife and I taught essential oils classes. Eventually I was asked by Young Living to teach about essential oils and psychology to groups of distributors in the US as well as in Asia. As I mentioned in the introduction, this is where I honed my skills and developed my ideas about how oils and psychology interact.

I began to feel torn, though. Different people were telling me that in order to excel at something, I needed to focus on one thing. People who knew me from the essential oils world encouraged me to focus on that in order to rise to the top of the ranks. That would be fine, except I loved my psychology work and I knew that it was an expression of what I was meant to do on earth. I considered dropping the essential oils teaching and just focusing on psychology, but that did not feel quite right either, because in the essential oil world, I had found a community of people who were empowering themselves with natural solutions to our modern health crises, and who had become valued friends.

I ended up speaking to one of my mentors, Connie Marie. She herself had been a high school teacher for many years before joining Young Living and rising to a high rank as a leader. She understood about living in "two worlds." I expressed my dilemma to her, how I felt I needed to focus, but that I did not want to cut off either of my two interests, psychology and essential oils. She thought about it for a minute, and then said to me: "Create a tool."

A light bulb went off at that moment, and I was able to see a path forward, and out of my dilemma. This concept was significant because one of the principles of teaching and education in Young Living is the concept of "duplication."

When you teach others what you know, the effect of this teaching is normally limited by the number of people you can reach at a time. However, if you can teach using a tool such as a book or a video, this media can be passed from person to person, or disseminated widely, and the total effect of your teaching is exponential. Thus, the key to helping lots of people is to condense what you know into a format that can be replicated.

So, one of the first questions I had as I began to write my book was, how to put what I did with clients into a step-by-step formula or recipe that could be duplicated by others. It was this motivation that led to the original formulation of the 12-step Aroma Freedom Technique process in 2016.

After the book came out, one of the most rewarding moments for me came when I received a phone call from someone who had found the book online. She was a massage therapist from Florida, and she told me that when she received the book in the mail, she immediately tried the 12-step process on herself. She said that she suffered from a skin condition that she knew had some relationship to her emotions, because it would always get worse when she was stressed. But she did not know which emotions were to blame. So, she did the process with the goal of clearing out any emotions that related to her skin condition. By following the steps, she found herself tapping into some deep feelings and memories that she did not expect. She smelled the oils as directed and noticed herself feeling calmer and more balanced. And, the next day, she noticed that her skin condition was about 80% better.

This was exciting news for me - not just because she had a great result, but because she had accomplished this feat without me! It was proof to me that the steps HAD duplicated my skills, and that the process of gaining emotional freedom using Aroma Freedom Technique could spread through the world via this teachable and duplicatable technique rather than through my individual, 1-1 attention with a client.

I mention all of this for two reasons. First, to point out that the concepts of teaching, self-empowerment, and helping others are baked into the origins of Aroma Freedom. These techniques are meant to be shared far and wide and used on yourself and others. My goal was, and still is, to enable people all over the world to benefit from these processes.

Second, to return to Young Living Essential Oils, I would like to explain a little more deeply why I recommend using them in the Aroma Freedom Processes. Yes, I have been a distributor of these oils for over 20 years, but I have not written this book and done all this work just to sell you some oils! If I was only looking to grow my Young Living business, this is not the path I would have taken.

My connection and dedication to Young Living arises from several areas.

1. The love and support we have received from the Young Living community since the very first day we joined has been nothing short of remarkable. We have had people guide us and connect us to the resources we needed, no matter what issues we were trying to solve, whether for ourselves or others.

2. The farms! Young Living is the only major Essential Oils company that owns and develops many of the farms used to grow the aromatic herbs that it distills into oils. Gary Young grew up on a farm in Idaho and spent years learning how to grow and distill these plants for maximal potency. Young Living members can tour the many farms all over the world, and even help with the planting and harvests!

3. The science. Young Living has a team of scientists and state of the art laboratories to be able to verify essential oil purity and efficacy. Essential Oils vary widely in their chemical constituents depending on where they were grown, how they were distilled, the type of seed, and most importantly, whether any chemicals were used to process or extend the oil. Young Living has strict standards for quality and rejects oils that do not meet these standards. No pesticides, herbicides, or GMO seeds are ever allowed. They are organic.

4. The founders. Gary and Mary Young are genuine,

hard-working, dedicated, brilliant, and caring people. We met them many times over the years, and I had the chance to speak with Gary on several occasions about essential oils for emotional healing. Gary studied all over the world and was one of the pioneers in re-introducing essential oils to the modern world.

5. The blends. Gary Young was masterful in blending oils to accomplish a specific purpose. He made blends for the immune system, the digestive system, the musculoskeletal system, and of course for the emotions. This is as much an art as a science, and when we use the blends he created, such as "Inner Child," "Trauma Life," or "Release," they stimulate the brain and the emotions in safe and predictable ways. These blends are not available from other companies.

6. The copycats. Following on the heels of the success of Young Living, there are many companies that have rushed in to offer "similar" oils at lower prices. There was even one company that split off from Young Living, copied many of their recipes, and tried to recruit Young Living members to their ranks. (I know this because they actually contacted me and my wife and invited us to join them, then later denied that they ever contacted any members.) Such behavior among other companies has made us wary of the claims that they have about their purity, and of course none of them know how to grow the plants. For this reason, we stick with a company that we have been with for 2 decades and have been consistent in their quality.

7. The efficacy and results. People are often surprised the first time they smell a Young Living essential oil - if they are used to perfume grade or mass-produced oils, they note that YL oils smell very "strong." And, when they apply them for various health and wellness conditions, they notice how quickly they see results. When combined with the specific psychological focusing techniques found in Aroma Freedom, the results are stunning. People are continually amazed at how quickly they feel better. This is due to the magic combination of Aroma Freedom and Young Living Oils.

For all these reasons, I only recommend Young Living oils for the Aroma Freedom processes. I am sure that there are other essential oils in the world that are high quality, organic, and come from companies with integrity - but I don't know which ones they are! For the sake of keeping with a standard that we know works, we exclusively use Young Living Essential Oils.

In order to become certified and to use them in your practice, you will need to get about a half a dozen of the YL oils + blends:

- Lavender
- Stress Away
- Frankincense
- Inner Child
- Release
- Transformation or Believe

Additional oils used can include:

- Clarity
- Trauma Life
- SARA
- Present Time
- Forgiveness
- Surrender

If you don't yet have an account, we can help you get the oils you need at www.aromafreedom.com/oils. If you already know a Young Living Distributor who sent you to this book, they can help you to get started.

A final word about the Essential Oils used in Aroma Freedom

Here is some additional information about the oils we use. Note that there is much more information available online, in books, and in many of the great courses and Aromatherapy certifications out there. My hope here is to whet your appetite to learn more and to do your own research - which is easier than ever with all of the online databases. If you would like a primer in how I do research, you may enjoy a class I did a few months back on the connection between essential oils and oxytocin - you can access the replay here: www.aromafreedom.com/research

Happy learning!

Lavender essential oil, often referred to as the "swiss army knife" of essential oils because of its versatility, is one of the most popular and beloved oils. Generally regarded as calming, it has been studied especially for its ability to help with insomnia, depression, stress relief, skin conditions, burn relief, acne, and antimicrobial activity.

In Aroma Freedom, we use lavender as part of the "Memory Release Blend," which includes lavender, frankincense, and Stress Away Blend. Lavender, in the form of a commercially available capsule (Sold as a pharmaceutical by prescription as "Silexan" in Germany, and available over the counter as "Calm Aid" in the USA) has been shown to be as effective as Valium in hundreds of research studies. It seems to work on the Serotonin and GABA systems in the body.

It is also one of the most commonly adulterated essential oils, and is sometimes sold in synthetic form (as a combination of linalool and linalyl acetate), or in its hybrid form (Lavandin), without proper labeling. Such use may lead to skin irritation or even burns. This is why care must be taken when choosing the source of essential oils used in Aroma Freedom.

Frankincense essential oil

Frankincense has been used for thousands of years for its ability to support physical, emotional, and spiritual wellness. An entire infrastructure of caravans, trading centers, port cities, and more was widespread in the ancient world primarily to facilitate the transport and delivery of Frankincense resin. It was valued higher than gold due to its utility and spiritual significance.

Modern science has validated the use of frankincense and its derivatives (such as incensole acetate) as containing anti-depressant and anti-anxiety properties. It has even been shown to activate a specific (TRPV3) channel in the brain that induces calming in ways that other compounds do not.

Although not fully understood, the use of frankincense resin in many religious traditions, including the Ancient Egyptian, Jewish, Roman, Greek, and Christian, suggests a significant psychoactive, if not spiritual, effect. I will propose that the use of such compounds as frankincense in religious rituals is motivated by the need to transport us away from the "stress and strain" of everyday life, and into a state of inner communion, wherein we can hear the voice of wisdom and guidance we seek. As we observe in all of the Aroma Freedom techniques, the reduction of emotional charge, whether for past, present, or future worries, is almost always experienced along with a "voice of wisdom" that speaks to us and gives us guidance and comfort.

A note about Essential Oil Blends:

The Blends referenced in this book were created by Dr. Gary Young, founder of Young Living Essential Oils over 30 years ago. He synthesized vast research about the chemistry of essential oils with his knowledge of growing, harvesting, and distilling aromatic herbs and his spiritual and scriptural understanding of oils to create these blends. Although Young Living gives us the ingredients of each blend, the exact proportions as well as the method of blending is proprietary. The ingredients below are for reference only and to help you in your own research about the amazing world of essential oils. Best results will be obtained by using the blends created by Young Living Essential Oils.

Contact us at www.aromafreedom.com/oils for help with ordering.

Stress Away Blend (From Young Living)

- Copaiba (Copaifera officinalis resin) oil.
- Lime (Citrus aurantifolia) oil.
- Cedarwood (Cedrus atlantica) bark oil.
- Vanilla (Vanilla planifolia) fruit extract.
- Ocotea (Ocotea quixos) leaf oil.
- Lavender (Lavandula angustifolia) oil.

Trauma Life Blend (From Young Living)

- Frankincense (Boswellia carteri) oil
- Sandalwood (Santalum album) oil
- Valerian (Valeriana officinalis) oil
- Lavender (Lavandula angustifolia) oil
- Davana (Artemisia pallens) oil
- Spruce (Picea mariana) oil
- Geranium (Pelargonium graveolens) oil
- Helichrysum (Helichrysum italicum) oil
- Kaffir Lime (Citrus hystrix) oil
- Rose (Rosa damascena) oil

Inner Child Blend (From Young Living)

- Orange (Citrus aurantium dulcis) oil
- Tangerine (Citrus reticulata) oil
- Ylang Ylang (Cananga odorata) oil
- Sandalwood (Santalum paniculatum) oil
- Jasmine (Jasminum officinale) absolute
- Lemongrass (Cymbopogon flexuosus) oil
- Spruce (Picea mariana) oil

- Bitter Orange (Citrus aurantium amara) oil

Release Blend (From Young Living)

- Ylang Ylang (Cananga odorata) oil
- Olive Fruit Oil
- Lavendin (Lavandula hybrida) oil
- Geranium (Pelargonium graveolens) oil
- Sandalwood (Santalum paniculatum) oil
- Grapefruit (Citrus paradisi) oil
- Tangerine (Citrus reticulata) oil
- Spearmint (Mentha Spicata) leaf extract
- Lemon (Citrus Limon) oil
- Blue Cypress (Calliotris intratropica) wood oil
- Davana (Artemisia pallens) flower oil
- Kaffir Lime (Citris hystrix) lead extract
- Ocotea (Ocotea quixos) leaf oil
- Jasmine (Jasminum officinale) absolute
- German Chamomile (Chamomilla recutita) flower oil
- Blue Tansy (Tanacetum annuum) flower oil
- Rose (Rosa damascena) flower oil

Clarity Blend (From Young Living)

- Basil (Ocimum basilicum) oil
- Cardamom seed (Elettaria cardamomum) oil
- Rosemary (Rosmarinus officinalis) oil
- Peppermint (Mentha piperita) oil
- Coriander seed (Coriandrum sativum) oil
- Geranium flower (Pelagonium graveolens) oil
- Bergamot peel (Citrus aurantium bergamia) oil

- Lemon peel (Citrus limon) oil
- Ylang Ylang flower (Cananga odorata) oil
- Jasmine (Jasminum officinale) absolute
- Roman Chamomile flower (Anthemis nobilis) oil
- Palmarosa (Cymbopogon martini) oil

Transformation Blend (From Young Living)

- Lemon peel (Citrus Limon) oil
- Peppermint (Mentha piperita) oil
- Sandalwood (Santalum paniculatum) oil
- Clary Sage (Salvia sclarea) oil
- Sacred Frankincense (Boswellia sacra) oil
- Idaho blue spruce (Picea pungens) oil
- Cardamom seed (Elettaria cardamomum) oil
- Ocotea (Ocotea quixos) oil
- Palo Santo (Bursera graveolens) oil

Believe Blend (From Young Living)

- Balsam Fir (Abies balsamea) oil
- Coriander seed (Coriandrum sativum) oil
- Bergamot (Citrus aurantium) oil
- Frankincense (Boswellia carterii) oil
- Idaho Blue Spruce (Picea pungens) oil
- Ylang Ylang flower (Cananga odorata) oil
- Geranium (Pelargonium graveolens) oil

Selected Essential Oil Research about oils in the Blends:

Copaiba essential oil is one of the highest known sources of beta caryophyllene, a potent anti-inflammatory compound. It has also been studied and found to contain an anti-anxiety action similar to Valium –
https://pubmed.ncbi.nlm.nih.gov/19703355/

Lime essential oil is uplifting, refreshing, and has been known to help with feelings of apathy.

Cedarwood essential oil tends to be mentally stimulating, and may have a positive effect on cognition and brain function. Biblical scholars note that King Solomon (known as the wisest king) built his entire temple from cedarwood. Scientists in Japan have found that inhaling cedarwood oil during monotonous work conditions had the effect of raising DHEA-S levels, a hormone that acts as a precursor to both Testosterone and Estrogen. This may be the mechanism by which it affects mood and cognition.
https://pubmed.ncbi.nlm.nih.gov/28117719/

Vanilla scent is one of the most universally favored aromas throughout the world, across many cultures. Scientists have discovered that smelling vanilla can raise the "pain threshold" of people with chronic pain.
https://pubmed.ncbi.nlm.nih.gov/32289824/ It is possible that reduction in physical pain and reduction in emotional pain, as seen in the effects of essential oils during Aroma Freedom, may follow similar pathways.

Ocotea essential oil has a scent like a mild cinnamon. It has been studied mostly for its role in blood sugar regulation, anti-inflammatory, antibiotic, antithrombotic, and antiplatelet activity. It is possible that the mild sweetness of the oil contributes to its emotional effect, but this has not yet been researched.

Sandalwood essential oil is another wood oil (along with frankincense, cedarwood, and various conifers, see below) that has had a long and storied use throughout history. It is a favorite incense in many religious and spiritual traditions, especially in India. Sandalwood oil has been shown to increase salivary oxytocin levels in post-menopausal women - https://pubmed.ncbi.nlm.nih.gov/32013535/. Oxytocin is a hormone that stimulates feelings of trust, attachment, bonding, and love. The ability of sandalwood to induce positive feelings plays an important role in recovering from trauma.

Many of our most significant traumas come from feelings of betrayal from those close to us - parents, siblings, romantic and life partners. When we have an "attachment wound," this can induce feelings of mistrust, anger, hurt, and shame. Sandalwood is a sweet and nurturing aroma that seems to help reverse this trend, especially when used within the context of the full Aroma Freedom protocols.

Valerian essential oil has a strong, musky scent, and has been studied extensively for its sleep inducing properties. https://pubmed.ncbi.nlm.nih.gov/35990355/ It seems to work by activating the serotonergic and GABA pathways. Additionally, its anti-anxiety effects are well known and thus help to shift the nervous system into a parasympathetic mode and away from the "fight and flight" reaction. This calming effect is important especially when processing intense emotions and memories.

Davana essential oil has been used in southern India for centuries but has only recently been studied scientifically. It has a unique quality of smelling differently on each person, due to its unique chemical makeup. Anecdotally it is an aphrodisiac, and there is some science supporting its use as an insect repellant https://pubmed.ncbi.nlm.nih.gov/26434107/, anti-inflammatory https://pubmed.ncbi.nlm.nih.gov/34669255/, and antioxidant https://www.ncbi.nlm.nih.gov/pmc/articles/PMC3103929/. It has a sweet and exotic aroma and is included in the Trauma Life blend to enhance feelings of joy and happiness.

Spruce essential oil is one of the best sources of polyprenols, which are compounds that have been studied for their anti-stress and anti-aging effects. It may help with the integrity of cell membranes, and with enhancing the effects of the other essential oils in the blend. Ropren, a pharmaceutical drug derived from polyprenols, has been studied for its anxiolytic and antidepressant effect as well - https://pubmed.ncbi.nlm.nih.gov/21086644/ .

Geranium essential oil is well known as a calming and soothing scent. It has been shown to increase alpha waves in female subjects - https://www.ncbi.nlm.nih.gov/pmc/articles/PMC9102723/ - and to help with both anxiety - https://pubmed.ncbi.nlm.nih.gov/29122262/ - and depression -

https://pubmed.ncbi.nlm.nih.gov/30236298/ - in clinical studies.

Helichrysum essential oil is a precious and difficult to obtain essential oil that has been used for centuries in traditional mediterranean medicine and folk healing. Recent studies highlight its powerful antimicrobial and antiinflammatory properties - https://pubmed.ncbi.nlm.nih.gov/34762977/. It also has been studied to assist with mental exhaustion and moderate burnout - https://pubmed.ncbi.nlm.nih.gov/23140115/. Unresolved emotional pain can be exhausting, and smelling this oil during the Aroma Freedom process can assist with giving you the energy to complete the journey with more ease.

Kaffir Lime essential oil has been studied for its antioxidant, anti inflammatory and metabolic enhancement effects - https://www.ncbi.nlm.nih.gov/pmc/articles/PMC8875002/

About the Author

Dr. Benjamin Perkus is a Licensed Psychologist who has pioneered the use of Aromatherapy for resolving traumatic and painful memories, and for developing the Aroma Freedom Technique to help people release their limitations and be empowered to realize their goals and dreams.

He has an undergraduate degree in Philosophy from Binghamton University, and a Doctorate in Psychology from Duquesne University, as well as many additional certifications and training in both Psychology and Aromatherapy. He has presented nationally and internationally at conferences and workshops.

His first book, "The Aroma Freedom Technique: Using Essential Oils to Transform your Emotions and Realize Your Heart's Desire" has inspired thousands of people to take control of their emotions, free themselves from painful memories, and pursue a life of passion and purpose.

Since that book's publication, he has certified hundreds of people in Aroma Freedom, and serves a large online community of students who have chosen to free themselves and others using these techniques.

In his spare time, he enjoys traveling, house and garden projects, spending time with his family, and of course learning and reading something every day.

To reach Dr. Perkus regarding speaking engagements, or for any other questions, he can be reached at:

ben@aromafreedom.com

or

Call/text our Aroma Freedom Hotline at 607-725-7785

www.ingramcontent.com/pod-product-compliance
Lightning Source LLC
Chambersburg PA
CBHW060243100426
42742CB00011B/1623